Assessing Asian Language Performance

Guidelines for Evaluating Limited-English-Proficient Students

Second Edition

Li-Rong Lilly Cheng, Ph.D.
Coordinator, Bilingual Multicultural Program
Department of Communicative Disorders
San Diego State University
San Diego, California

Foreword by Katharine G. Butler, Ph.D.
Director, Center for Research
Syracuse University
Syracuse, New York

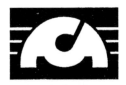
**Academic
Communication
Associates, Inc.**

P.O. Box 4279
Oceanside, California 92052-4279

Assessing Asian Language Performance
Second Edition
Copyright © 1991 by Academic Communication Associates.

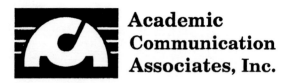 Academic
Communication
Associates, Inc.

P.O. Box 4279
Oceanside, California 92052-4279

Toll-Free Telephone Number for Book Orders: (888) 758-9558
WEB: http://www.acadcom.com
E-Mail: acom@acadcom.com
Printed in the United States of America
Library of Congress Catalog Card No: 90-85887
International Standard Book Number: 0-930951-47-6

Assessing Asian Language Performance is a
volume in Academic Communication Associates'

Multicultural Special Education Series

Practical resources designed to help educational professionals
provide appropriate instructional programs for students
from diverse cultural and linguistic backgrounds

Table of Contents

Foreword

For several decades, there has been an escalating concern in education to identify appropriate assessment measures for evaluating minority children. While the public is most widely accustomed to reading about the possible bias of intelligence tests (Hilliard, 1987), it is the verbal aspects of intelligence that are seen as being unfair to those with differing social, cultural, and linguistic backgrounds. Speech-language pathologists, psychologists, bilingual educators, among others, recognize that it is often difficult to separate the language status of a child from his or her academic performance. Riles (1987) makes an interesting point about the use of intelligence and other tests:

> In my view, no test is comprehensive enough in itself for one to make a sweeping judgment about an individual's potential. The problem is that tests are sometimes misused. But, if you ban the use of the I.Q. test because it has been misused, the same logic follows for any other test. And if all tests are banned, we would be left only with the judgment of the teacher, which in many cases is more insensitive and prejudicial than the tests themselves.
>
> (Riles, 1987, pp. 20, 28)

Assessment, therefore, is an act that cannot be undertaken lightly, whether it be for the purposes of establishing an intelligence quotient, or for establishing a language difference or disorder. Using language to assess language requires special skill under the best of circumstances. It requires even greater understanding and knowledge if one seeks to differentiate between the presence of a dialect or the presence of a disorder, the degree of language competency present in first and second language acquisition, and the possible interrelationship between language proficiency and academic success.

As Riles (1987) suggests, teacher judgment is frequently questioned when placement decisions are under scrutiny. That monolingual professionals without understanding or knowledge of other cultures can make significant errors is indisputable. Errors can also occur if there is insufficient understanding of the linguistic nature of the child's first language. Dr. Cheng, the author of this text, has attempted to right these two wrongs. Underlying the entire volume is the theme of cultural constraints and linguistic differences. Utilizing that theme, Cheng assists the reader to gain insight into a number of Asian cultures and a detailed understanding of linguistic similarities and differences. Even more importantly, she offers a variety of procedures and methods by which a monolingual English speaker may conduct assessment and intervention with children whose backgrounds and first language represent one of the Asian rim countries.

Recognizing the inherent difficulty of evaluating a child who is of Limited English Proficiency (LEP) or is non-English Speaking (NES), Cheng identifies a team approach to assessment that can circumvent some of the problems that have been identified. While it is generally conceded that children should be evaluated by a trained professional who speaks the child's first language, there is an overwhelming shortage of multilingual professionals. For example only 1% of the 50,000 members of the American Speech-Language-Hearing Association are proficient enough in a foreign language to provide clinical services to foreign language speakers and an infinitesimal number who are proficient in any of the Asian languages. Yet Asian immigrants and refugees are to be found in each of the 50 states, and the territories of Guam and Puerto Rico. According to Walker (1985, p.54), Southeast Asian refugees are joining "a rapidly increasing Asian American population. Americans of Asian and Pacific Island origin have increased 120 percent since 1972, and number 1.5 percent of the total population."

Since 1975, 700,000 Southeast Asian immigrants have come to the United States, with the majority of them being Vietnamese, followed by Laotians and Cambodians. There are vivid cultural, as well as linguistic differences, between many Asian countries and the United States. Since some Asian languages are tonal in nature, characterized by pitch changes within a word that affects lexical meaning, monolingual speakers of English have considerable difficulty in assessing speakers of tonal languages, where the use of an incorrect tone results in a mispronunciation or the saying of an entirely different word from the one intended. Throughout the book, Dr. Cheng addresses such differences, identifying the "language families" of a number of different languages. As she points out, some of them are logographic, others alphabetic; some are tonal, others not; some are inflectional, others not; some are essentially monosyllabic, others not. Throughout the various chapters, Cheng provides massive amounts of information that assist in defining the possible phonetic interferences stemming from Asian language knowledge to the acquisition of English.

While *Assessing Asian Language Performance* focuses upon the comprehension and production of spoken language, the possibility of using samples of written Asian languages is explored. While in the U.S. we speak of "breaking the English code" as essential to reading, e.g., a sound-symbol correspondence, there are different parameters for breaking the code in Asian languages. For example, Foorman (1986) points out that Japanese children learn to read utilizing both the syllabic code of kana and the morphographic code of kanji, thus providing the fluent Japanese reader with four internal codes for a word: kanji, kana, phonetic, and meaning-based. Cheng discusses some of the differences and similarities of Japanese and Chinese, and also dwells upon the cultural aspects of these two populations in terms of family and community relationships. Cheng's efforts to identify crucial cultural constraints and the mismatch between educational expectations of parents and children are well taken, since both Asian parents and children, based on prior experience, expect American schools to be much more structured and formal. Evidence of Cheng's position may be found in a 1984 study by Lee, Stigler and Stevenson who studied 13,221 first graders in Minneapolis and Taipei. On equivalent forms of a test in both Chinese and English, they found that Chinese children at age 6 read with significantly more ease. The authors attributed the results to (1) the parental belief systems, (2) children's attendance to tasks while in the classroom, and (3) the amount of homework completed by each group. For example, few Chinese mothers were satisfied with their child's academic performance, while American mothers appeared to be very positive, even though their children performed less well. "These data pose an interesting paradox. American mothers were more positive than the Chinese mothers about their children's scholastic experiences and progress. At the same time, the American children generally demonstrated lower levels of achievement in reading." (Lee, Stigler, & Stevenson, 1984, p. 148). The authors also report that they found strong evidence that Chinese children listened to their teacher and attended to task demands much more frequently than American children, who tended to talk to their peers, asked inappropriate or irrelevant questions, wandered around the room, and so forth. Finally, the authors reported that American parents and teachers did not appear to consider homework to be of great value, in marked contrast to Chinese parents and teachers. A survey of mothers' time estimates of at-home study were 14 minutes per day on weekdays, 3 minutes on Saturday, and 4 minutes on Sunday for the American first graders, and 77 minutes each weekday, 66 minutes on Saturday, and 42 minutes on Sunday for the Chinese children. This study would appear to underscore Cheng's comments on the difficulty that Asian children experience in adjusting to American schools and American teachers.

Cheng addresses the need to assess Asian children in both their first and second language, and amply demonstrates the usefulness of interpreters and translators in reaching an understanding of the linguistic and cultural fabric of the child's verbal and nonverbal behavior in the context of the family and of the school. The importance of using an ecologically valid system of language assessment is stressed throughout the various chapters, along with a system for measuring language proficiency that is remarkable in its depth.

Wisely, Cheng has recommended a team approach, using not only interpreters but bilingual teachers and aides, parents, community representatives, and others. She provides a host of suggestions so that even monolingual personnel can use observation, consultation, and assessment instruments to evaluate the communicative competence of children in their first and second language. The use of careful observation and consultation is also stressed in both formal and informal settings. Cheng, who speaks a number of Asian and European languages, is a linguist who understands her subject. Coming to the U.S. by way of Shanghai and Taiwan, her training as a speech-language pathologist and bilingual educator permit her to share her insights with the reader. Her familiarity with the cultures and languages of the Asian rim countries pervades each chapter.

On a happy note, Cheng stresses that although one may be unable to speak the language of the Asian minority client, the speech-language pathologist who is trained in language acquisition and language disorders can assess and remediate language disorders in Asian children through a team approach that utilizes interpreters, informants, bilingual educators, careful assessment in both languages, and a careful attention to the functional nature of communicative competence in multiple contexts.

Of considerable value to the reader are the instruments, both formal and informal, that are provided throughout the text: behavioral assessment protocols, articulation tests in various languages, language elicitation procedures, a communication checklist, indicators of pragmatic competence, and so forth. These are valuable additions to the test armanentarium of the speech-language pathologist, psychologist, or bilingual educator.

While it may well take expert assessment skills to identify the specific point on the continuum of language learning when the child may require language intervention (in the clinical sense) rather than language instruction (Butler, 1985), this book provides much needed direction to the search for appropriate methods and procedures.

In summary, while identification of a language disorder in a first or second language remains a cloudy assessment issue, Cheng has shed considerable light on a very knotty problem. This book may well serve as a seminal contribution to the literature in language assessment and intervention with limited-English-proficient Asian minority students.

Katharine G. Butler, PhD
Director, Center for Research
Syracuse University

REFERENCES

Butler, K.G./From the editor. Language 1 and language 2: Implications for language disorders. *Topics in Language Disorders*, 5:4, p. vi.

Foorman, B.R. (1986). Non-alphabetic codes in learning to read: the case of the Japanese. In B.R. Foorman and A.W. Siegel (Eds.), *Acquisition of reading skills: Cultural constraints and cognitive universals* (pp. 115–122). Hillsdale, NJ: Lawrence Erlbaum Associates.

Hilliard, A.G. (1987). Conflicting ideas on the banning of intelligence tests: Commentary. *Education Week*, February 11, pp. 20, 28.

Lee, S., Stigler, J.W., & Stevenson, H.W. (1986). Beginning reading in Chinese and English. In B.R. Foorman & A.W. Siegel (Eds.), *Acquisition of reading skills: cultural constraints and cognitive universals*, (pp. 123–150). Hillsdale, NJ: Lawrence Erlbaum Associates.

Riles, W.R. (1987). Conflicting ideas on the banning of intelligence tests: Commentary. *Education Week*, February 11, pp. 20, 28.

Walker, C.L. (1985). Learning English: the Southeast Asian refugee experience, *Topics in Language Disorders*, 5:4.

Preface

In recent years, there has been an influx of Asian/Pacific Islander (API) immigrants and refugees into the United States. Yet, there is an extreme shortage of trained speech-language clinicians who are able to speak any of the Asian languages or languages spoken in the Pacific Islands. Recent surveys conducted by the American Speech-Language-Hearing Association (ASHA) provide evidence that many of the Asian languages are not spoken by any of its members. Although a few speech-language pathologists speak Chinese or Japanese, no ASHA members reported being fluent in Khmer, Laotian, Hmong, Yiu-Mienh, Thai, Indonesian, Burmese, Korean, or any of the Filipino languages.

The primary purpose of this book is to provide information about the cultural and linguistic characteristics of the API language minorities and to suggest innovative assessment and intervention strategies for speech-language clinicians and other language specialists who work with these groups. The book includes critical background information about the API language minority populations in the United States and the various cultures of Asia. The book also includes descriptions of the linguistic systems of the API languages and a contrastive analysis showing how these languages vary from English. Such information is an essential part of the pre-assessment process.

Many Asian immigrants and refugees have experienced severe adjustment problems because of their linguistic and cultural differences. They are unfamiliar with the choice of foods, the way of cooking, the tools of cooking, the way of schooling, the choice of clothing, the various forms of transportation, and even the use of the toilet. To them, food processors, toasters, microwave ovens, and can openers are foreign objects. Daily, they are confounded by the newness of the environment and the high technology of the United States. It is understandable that many feel a sense of alienation and dislocation.

Immigrants from Asia and the Pacific Islands represent diverse cultural, linguistic, and religious backgrounds. They are Buddhists, Moslems, Taoists, Shintoists, Catholics, and Protestants. Some practice herbal medicine, and some practice folk medicine. Some are preliterate, and some are literate. Some are highly educated, and some have never been in school. Some are multilingual, and some are monolingual. Some come from rural areas, and some come from metropolitan centers.

Many of the Asian languages come from different language "families." Some of the Asian languages are logographic; some are alphabetic. Some of the Asian languages are tonal; others are not. Some are inflectional; others are noninflectional. Some of them use the system of agglutination; others do not. Some of the languages are essentially monosyllabic; others are polysyllabic.

Although the Asian languages vary greatly, the Asian people have many cultural commonalities that provide not only a sense of kinship among them, but also a shared context for their use of language. Furthermore, there are many commonalities in the nonverbal, paralinguistic communication of the Asian language minorities. It is imperative, therefore, that monolingual English-speaking language specialists attempt to understand the Asian cultures and identify the reasons for certain proxemic, kinesic, and pragmatic forms of communication among the Asian language minorities.

Speech, language, and hearing professionals must cultivate their sensitivity and awareness of cultural differences and social setting constraints in Asian learning styles in order to make the adjustments necessary to meet the needs of the Asian language minority students. They must provide opportunities for Asian language minority students to develop their English verbal skills, "tailor" the activities to accommodate the students' experience and culture, and lead them to discovery and problem solving. Because it is unlikely that the United States will have many trained language professionals who can speak the various Asian languages for several years to come, monolingual speech-language pathologists must accept the responsibility for providing adequate language assessment and intervention services to these students. As there are almost no reliable professional resources, monolingual English-speaking speech-language clinicians must develop a sense of resourcefulness and confidence to meet the needs of these students, be flexible and observant during assessment and intervention, be open-minded and sensitive to the needs of these children, and finally, be aware of multicultural, multilingual differences. I hope that reading this book will lead speech-language clinicians through a self-discovery process whereby they become more understanding and empathic toward Asian language minorities, more flexible about their own views, and, most important, more accepting of cultural and linguistic commonalities and differences.

Acknowledgments

So many individuals contributed directly or indirectly to the production of the first and second editions of this book that it is impossible to thank them individually. I have been particularly inspired by Dr. Katharine Butler who provided me with endless support, continuous guidance, and critical suggestions.

I am also indebted to my "natural support system"— my entire family, without whose understanding, this book could never have been completed. My special thanks go to Kenneth Tom, who edited the first draft of the manuscript. I would like to thank Caroline Fung, a talented artist, for the new illustrations that have been added to the second edition of this book. In addition, I wish to thank the reviewers and the entire editorial support staff.

Finally, I want to thank the children and their parents who have allowed me into their world and have shared their personal life histories. I have learned so much from them and have confirmed the belief that we need to let the children lead the way, to engage their parents in the educational process, and to utilize their natural support system in our service delivery. It is through the collective wisdom of the concerned and dedicated individuals that we can hope for a better and brighter future for all.

L. C.

PART I

Critical Background Information: The Asian Language Minorities in the United States

CHAPTER 1

Asian Cultural and Linguistic Values

A precise, inclusive definition of culture has eluded humankind for centuries. In 1871, Tylor included the following elements in his definition of culture: knowledge, belief, art, morals, law, custom, and any other capabilities and habits acquired by people as members of society. When two anthropologists, Kroeber and Kluckhohn (1954), examined more than 300 such definitions of culture, they still could not find a satisfactory definition. It is difficult to define culture in a narrow sense, because culture itself is such a broad concept (i.e., "the ways of a people"). It encompasses all aspects of human life and the patterns for living.

Culture is a system of standards for perceiving, believing, evaluating, and acting; it is composed of behavior patterns, symbols, institutional values, and other man-made elements of society. Brooks (1968) identified five aspects of culture: (1) biological growth, (2) personal refinement, (3) literature and the fine arts, (4) patterns of living, and (5) the sum total of a way of life. Kluckhohn and Kelly (1945) defined culture as "all those historically created designs for living, explicit and implicit, rational, irrational, and nonrational, which exist at any given time as potential guides for the behavior of men" (p. 554).

Kroeber (1952) described four qualities of culture:

1. It is transmitted and continued not by the genetic mechanism of heredity, but by interconditioning of zygotes.
2. Whatever its origins, culture quickly tends to become suprapersonal and anonymous.
3. It falls into patterns, or regularities of form, style, and significance.
4. It embodies values that may be formulated (overtly, as mores) or felt (covertly, as folkways) by the members of society.

Kroeber further stated that culture exists only when there is a society of individuals to share it. Conversely, every human society is accompanied by a culture.

The United Nations Educational, Scientific, and Cultural Organization (UNESCO; 1977) noted that culture is essentially a dynamic value system of learned attitudes, with assumptions, conventions, beliefs, and rules that permit members of a group to relate to each other and to the world. Similarly, Taylor (1986) defined culture as "the set of perceptions, technologies, survival systems used by members of a specified group to ensure the acquisition and perpetuation of what they consider to be a high quality of life'' (p. 2).

Anthropologists agree that patterns of culture are organized or structured into a system or set of systems that is subject to constant change (Lado, 1957). Boas (1946), in examining the element of change in culture, made the observation that collecting available data makes it possible to see ''changing cultures and local types developing here and there, inner developments and foreign elements giving rise to new forms'' (p. 668). All cultures go through varying degrees of change, depending on the extent of their contact with other cultures. The more frequently the culture has contact with the outside world, the more rapidly changes occur. These changes are clearly perceived by individuals who have left their culture for a number of years, adapted to another culture, and returned for a visit.

Culture is dynamic, never fixed or static; is learned and shared by a people; is creative and meaningful to the lives of individuals; is symbolically represented through the interactions of people; is governed by rules; has value and belief systems that guide people in their thinking, feeling, and acting; and is a continuous and cumulative process. In short, culture is the total way of life of people in a society.

Approaches to the Study of Culture

There are four different ways to examine cultures: (1) the emic view (inside), (2) the etic view (outside), (3) the fixed view, and (4) the dynamic view. The emic view is an examination of a culture from the perspective of a member of that culture and allows for an in-depth and qualitative understanding of cultural meanings and the origin of those meanings. Anthropologists such as Frake (1964) have used the emic approach to study cultures ''to account for the behavior of a people by describing the socially acquired and shared knowledge, or culture, that enables members of the society to behave in ways deemed appropriate by their fellows'' (p. 132). The etic view is an examination of a culture from the perspective of one who is not a member of that culture and allows for a fresh and comparative understanding of the culture. For example, a giggle may be interpreted as a sign of embarrassment by an Asian (the emic view), but as a sign of amusement by an American (the etic view).

The fixed view (i.e., the synchronic view) provides a description of a culture at a particular point in time and allows study of the structure, function, and meaning of a culture. In contrast, the dynamic view (i.e., the diachronic view) provides an understanding of a culture through its historical development and allows a comparison of different influences that may bring about cultural changes.

A combination of all these views produces a holistic approach to the study of a culture's four different aspects:

1. *the ideal:* that which people believe they do or ought to do as expressed in proverbs, stories, myths, jokes, rituals, and conversation
2. *the real:* the actual behavior of people as expressed in acts of deviation, failure, or complaints
3. *the explicit:* the observable, concrete, and consciously known elements of a culture as recognized in

- food
- fashion (e.g., style of dress, costumes)
- forms of language, historical to present
- facts and figures
- famous people
- folklore
- types of housing
- use of tools

4. *the implicit:* the invisible, silent, and unconscious elements of a culture as expressed in
   - values
   - attitudes
   - religious and spiritual beliefs
   - fears
   - kinship system
   - family structure
   - meaning of language

By their very nature, the implicit elements of a culture are difficult to define. Nonetheless, they are inherently part of a person's being and are reflected in that person's actions and thoughts. The values are unconsciously acquired, molded by the significant others in the person's life and personal experiences. For example, in an Asian culture, it is not uncommon for adults in their late 20s to maintain their emotional and economic dependence on their parents. If a family member were born handicapped or became physically or mentally handicapped, the Asian family would also take full responsibility for that person. Those in another culture may have very different attitudes about dependence and independence, however. Cross-cultural studies and attempts to understand people's attitudes make it possible to catch a glimpse of the implicit elements of cultures.

Cultural Conflict

There are more than 500 cultures in the United States. In the Southwest alone, there are more than 50 culturally and linguistically diverse societies. In the Los Angeles County area, speech-language services are provided to 88 different language groups. Taylor (1977), Taylor and Payne (1983), and Wolfram (1976) have all discussed the intercultural dimensions of the delivery of services to such a diverse population. They have asserted that clinicians must maintain a cross-cultural perspective in providing services. Taylor (1986) provided a model of the cultural interplay in everyday clinical encounters (Figure 1-1).

When two or more cultures come into contact with one another, conflicts may arise. For example, members of one culture may place great value on age, while members of the other may place great value on youth. The culture conflicts that occur when cultures come into contact may be either negative or positive. Negative conflict may result in

- culture shock
- marginality (a feeling of isolation one has when one remains on the margins of two cultures)

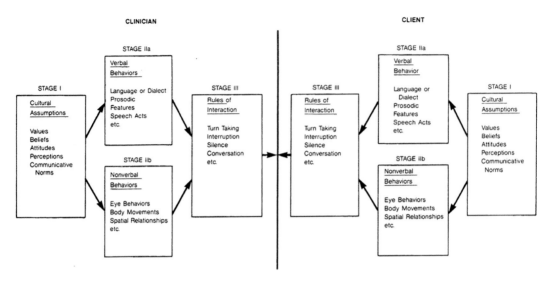

Figure 1-1 Cultural Interplay in Clinical Encounters

Source: From *Communication Disorders in Multicultural Populations* (p. 3) by L. Cole and V. Deal (Eds.), 1987, Rockville, Md.: American Speech-Language-Hearing Association. Copyright 1987 by American Speech-Language-Hearing Association. Reprinted by permission.

- bicultural confusion
- behaviors such as fighting, drinking, disrespect.

Positive conflict may bring about

- contrast and comparison
- innovation and change
- new strategies for survival
- behaviors that arise from a clear understanding of cultural values and from active rather than passive participation in cultural interaction

The history of the Chinese in America demonstrates the conflicts of cultures, their significance, and the acculturation process (McCunn, 1979). The first generation (19th century) of Chinese immigrants could not legally establish families in the United States. Also legally forbidden to socialize with non-Chinese, they saw little reason to learn Western customs or to learn more than a minimal amount of English. Calling them the "Yellow Peril" and the "Chinese Menace," U.S. workers wanted to force them out of the country. At the turn of the 20th century, some of the Chinese brought their families to the United States. Their children learned English by going to segregated American schools during the day; they learned Chinese by attending Chinese schools at night. As adults, these children generally maintained their home culture in isolated Chinatown neighborhoods. Chinatowns have grown and changed since the arrival of wives and families in the 1940s. The second and third generation Chinese-Americans who have become acculturated with life in the United States leave the confines of the Chinatowns to become a part of the larger American society. The degree of acculturation varies greatly among people in different areas, however.

Although variations in culture influence behavior; world view; thoughts; cognitive style; learning style; communicative style; human relational style; and the forms, content, and use of language, people from different cultures share similar thought processes. For example, everyone thinks about food when hungry; cultural differences appear in the kind of food that comes to mind. A Chinese may well envision a bowl of rice, while an American may think of a hamburger. A cross-cultural perspective makes it possible to learn through comparison and contrast, to increase mutual understanding, and to avoid areas of conflict.

Sapir stated that "all cultural behavior is patterned" (cited in Mandelbaum, 1949, p. 546). The rules may differ from one culture to another and from one language to another, however, and the same behavior (form) may have different meanings. For example, Spaniards view a bullfight as an art form, while people from a different culture may view it as an act of brutality against a defenseless animal. Similarly, the same behavior (form) may have different uses. For example, beans are served as salad in the United States, while beans are served only as dessert in some Asian countries.

A century ago, Spencer (1888) suggested that cultures are not isolated, but interdependent and that analysis of cultural traits often leads to faulty identification of diverse phenomena. Researchers need to be aware of cultural and linguistic relativity when studying cultures. It is essential to build respect for cultural differences and appreciation for cultural similarities.

Cultural Relativity

Cultural belief systems may differ slightly, or they may differ a great deal. Major differences in belief systems are sources of conflict. The following statements represent the beliefs of various societies and are the basis for the behavior of members of those societies:

- One should wear white to a funeral.
- One should not wear white to a wedding.
- Little boys wear blue; little girls wear pink.
- Black cats bring bad luck.
- Number four brings bad luck.
- Getting one's hair wet causes sickness.

There are many cultural ways that are correct and appropriate, each in its own sociocultural location and context. For example, Americans eat lettuce raw; the Chinese cook it. The two ways of eating lettuce are entirely different, but each is enjoyed by the people accustomed to eating lettuce in that way. Sometimes, a behavior that is considered appropriate in one culture may not be considered appropriate in another. For example, the Japanese consider burping a sign of appreciation for the food, yet Americans consider it ill-mannered to burp in public and excuse themselves after burping. The concept of cultural relativity helps people to develop a sense of tolerance for other cultures, to understand the many differences and similarities, and to avoid areas of culture conflict.

Linguistic Relativity

Researchers from different disciplines have long agreed that language is part of culture. Sixty years ago, Sapir (1921) recognized the intimate relationship between the content of language and culture. Although the form of language is explicit, the content and use of language may be implicit and may require interpretation in their cultural context—especially when people from different cultures use the same language.

Lexical items originate in the specific needs of people from a certain culture and reflect the unique way of life of those people. Labels define and differentiate concepts, phenomena, and objects that are vitally important to a culture. Thus, it is no surprise to find that the Eskimos have seven labels in their language for snow in its various forms, because snow is an important part of their way of life. Similarly, the Hawaiians have many words for coconut. Another example is beef, which is a staple of the American diet. There are many English words to describe the different cuts of beef (e.g., shank, T bone, rump roast, New York steak, Porterhouse steak). There is only one word for dish in Chinese, while there are as many as five words for dish in English, including plate, saucer, and platter. There are many words in Vietnamese to express the English word *carry*, however. For example, cầm means carry by hand; mang means carry in a pocket; ẵm means carry in the arms; ôm means carry tightly; đôi means carry on the head; cong means carry a human on the back; and gánh means carry a pole. In Vietnamese, the word *tủ* is used to mean bookshelf, cupboard, closet, box, refrigerator, cabinet, store window, and safe.

In the Asian cultures, the aged and the learned are revered. These people, as well as others with high social or family status, are addressed in special ways. In Vietnamese, there are more than 12 words for I or you; in Japanese, there are more than 100 words for I; and in Chinese, there are more than ten words for I. The rules for addressing people vary from language to language and from social context to social context. In Chinese, the family name is spoken first and the given name last. In Vietnamese, the first name is used after Mr., Mrs., or Miss. In Japanese, the word *san* is used after the name to show respect. In America, however, people often address each other by their first names.

Languages also have different semantic features. The word *yes* may mean no in Chinese, for example; a Vietnamese, who is asked, "Do you understand it?" may say "yes" meaning no, in order to save face. Consequently, the yes is a cultural yes, but a semantic no. This usage of yes in Chinese and Vietnamese may cause some problems in communication with Americans.

Pragmatic and paralinguistic rules differ from culture to culture. The accepted ways to sit or stand, as well as the distance that should be maintained between individuals, may vary greatly. The same gesture may mean different things in different cultures, causing difficulty in communication. For example, the American gesture used to beckon someone is the same as the Filipino gesture to wave good-bye. A Chinese who nods is not saying "yes," but simply "I hear you." When greeting someone, a Vietnamese may use the greeting "How is your health?"; a Chinese may use "Have you eaten?"; and a Filipino may ask "How are you?" and then "Have you eaten?" An Asian instructor views a student's silence as a sign of respect; an American instructor may interpret such a silence as a sign of passivity or a lack of interest.

There are also phonological, morphological, and syntactical differences in languages. For example, tense markers are an integral part of the English language, but no such markers exist in Thai or Tagalog. The morpheme /-s/ is used as a marker for plurality in English, but there is no such marker in Chinese. On the other hand, Chinese has unique functive verbs and resultative verbs to categorize parts of speech (Chang & Chang, 1978). Although there is no past tense marker in Vietnamese, people are capable of describing the past since the concept of past is shared by all people.

Comparison and contrast of any two linguistic systems provides a sense of linguistic relativity and an appreciation for both the similarities and the differences.

Assimilation and Cultural Pluralism

All those who wish to immigrate to the United States apply at the U.S. Department of Naturalization and Immigration. Some applicants are granted permanent resident status because they possess special skills; others, because family members petition for them. Some wait 6 years to receive their entry permit; others wait even longer, until a new quota is established.

Voluntary immigrants and refugees differ greatly in their motivation for emigration from their country of origin and the circumstances under which they emigrate (Davie, 1947; Garkovitch, 1977). Voluntary immigrants are generally prepared for their move. They are psychologically motivated and look forward to joining their families or to taking on new occupational challenges. In contrast, refugees are forced to leave their country of origin because of adverse domestic, social, or political conditions. They do not have the luxuries of planning or psychological preparation for immigration. As a result, the effects of culture shock on refugees are even more pervasive than are those on voluntary immigrants, and refugees may achieve lower levels of assimilation into their host country's society. All resettled immigrants tend to experience changes in cultural patterns in the course of adaptation, however, regardless of the motivation behind their emigration, (Davie, 1947; Gordon, 1964; Kent, 1953; Warner, 1945).

The United States has absorbed immigrants who came from all corners of the world, bringing with them different cultural values, religious beliefs, and languages. As a result, philosophers, sociologists, anthropologists, historians, religious leaders, and political leaders have long debated the ideal social structure for American society. The most popular theory of assimilation in the first decades of the 20th century required the Americanization of the new immigrants. Krug (1976) said that

> what the immigrants had to do was to shed, as quickly as possible, the cultural mores, political beliefs, modes of behavior, dress, various languages, eating habits, and to accept the evolved American culture and the ways of the American political democracy. (p. 6)

The supporters of Americanization shared a sense of ethnocentrism, believing that the Anglo-Saxon race was a superior race. They expected the immigrants from the "inferior" cultures to abandon their heritage and to live and behave as American Anglo-Saxons.

Grant (1919), the most outspoken in his time about the hereditary "superiority" of the Anglo-Saxon race, emphasized the need to preserve racial purity. He wrote,

> the results of the mixture of two races, in the long run, gives us a race reverting to the more ancient generalized and lower type . . . the cross between a white man and an Indian is an Indian, the cross between any of the three European races and a Jew is a Jew. (p. 16)

Boas (1946) voiced a very different opinion and maintained that the "existence of any pure race with special endowments is a myth, as is the belief that there are races all of whose members are foredoomed to eternal inferiority" (p. 106). Boas envisioned the total disappearance of the ethnic groups by mixed marriages. Although hundreds of thousands of immigrants did cut their ethnic ties, changed their names, and adopted the American culture, many others rejected the concept of Americanization, and the theory of the "melting pot" was born.

Unlike those who supported the theory of Americanization, those who supported the theory of the melting pot assumed that American culture was still in the process of being formed. They believed that all cultures should be fused, resulting in a new, superior American culture.

Neither the Americanization nor the melting pot theory applied to the Blacks, Mexican-Americans, Asian-Americans, or any other non-white immigrants or citizens, as their distinct appearances made it easy to differentiate them from Anglo-Americans. Seeing a need for a new theory, Kallen (1924) developed the theory of cultural pluralism. Kallen's main thesis was that American culture was not monolithic, but pluralistic, because "individuals move in and out freely from group to group, from home to the business or work or firm, or church, or political organization" (1956, p. 55). Kallen did not discuss the place of Blacks, Asians, Latinos, and other racial minorities in American culture, although he said that "all immigrants and their offspring are by the way undergoing 'Americanization' if they remain in one place in the country long enough, say six or seven years" (p. 79). Krug (1976) concluded that

> cultural pluralism, as originally defined by Horace Kallen, but broadened to include Blacks, Mexican Americans and the Spanish speaking groups, and Asian Americans may provide a new conceptual framework for the eventual mutually beneficial coexistence of the dominant American society and the various ethnic and racial minority groups. (p. 28)

Since the publication of Kallen's first book on cultural pluralism in 1924, many scholars have struggled with the dilemma of the relationship between the general American society (more specifically, the Anglo-American Protestant component) and the various ethnic and social minority groups. Gordon (1978) introduced the concept of structural pluralism and argued that ethnic groups are culturally assimilated into the Anglo-American society, but have separate ethnic subsocieties (e.g., Jewish social clubs, Chicano theaters, and Chinatowns). He believed that American society experienced a multiple acculturation, rather than a unidirectional cultural assimilation.

Banks (1979) described four levels of cross-cultural functioning:

1. superficial and brief cross-cultural encounters, such as eating in a restaurant that features food from another culture
2. more meaningful cross-cultural contacts and communications with members of other ethnic and cultural groups
3. ability to function comfortably in two different cultures
4. complete resocialization in another culture in terms of behavior, attitudes, and perceptions

Monolingual speech-language pathologists who work with the bilingual/multicultural population can become more comfortable with this group by cultivating their awareness of other cultures and peoples. Furthermore, as the language minority groups become acculturated, they will become more comfortable in communicating with the mainstream population. The degree of acculturation can be viewed as a continuum, and as one moves from one end to the other, one becomes more acculturated.

Education of Bilingual/Bicultural Children

In the early part of the 20th century, teachers considered bilingualism a liability, rather than an asset, because they felt that bilingualism caused confusion in children's cognitive development and delayed their linguistic development. Most teachers agreed that it was necessary to eradicate students' bilingualism if they were to be successful academically. Thus, children were punished for speaking their first language in school and made to feel ashamed of their own linguistic and cultural background.

The values from the home culture were often in conflict with those of the majority culture, making it difficult for the children to function adequately and appropriately. Many rejected their home culture, yet they were not accepted into the mainstream culture. They could not fit into either the majority or the minority culture, resulting in identity problems and marginality. Such conflict and confusion is real, and children from minority cultures may experience such difficulties even today. Ideally, these children should be viewed as people of complexity, not people of deficiency.

The recent influx of Chinese and Indochinese immigrants and refugees present more challenges for those who work with them. A clear and thorough understanding of their cultural background makes the provision of services a positive and productive experience for everyone.

Adjustments and Conflicts

There are vast individual differences in the educational and occupational backgrounds of Indochinese refugees, but their children are all likely to encounter certain adjustment problems and cultural conflicts. Wei (1983) discussed the three general areas of conflict that refugee children may face: (1) emotional, (2) cultural-social, and (3) educational.

Emotional Adjustments and Conflicts

The war in Vietnam left psychological scars on everyone who was a part of it and everyone who witnessed it. Many have been affected by the war to the extent that they have become emotionally unstable. Refugees not only were uprooted, but also were unprepared for life in the United States. During their evacuation or escape, many refugees experienced separation from their families, danger, deprivation, and starvation. All faced the uncertainties of the future. Some became cynical and distrustful, and all experienced culture shock when they first arrived in the United States.

Cultural-Social Adjustments and Conflicts

The first and most important barrier that faces refugee children is their inability to communicate in the English language. They cannot read street signs, directions, or any written materials. They cannot understand what people are saying. They observe unfamiliar items everywhere (e.g., in food, clothing, housing, transportation, and utensils), but cannot ask questions about their use. It takes a long time to solve such problems.

The Indochinese refugees are also confused about the different roles that they must play in their families. In Asian countries, the family is usually an extended one, often including three or four generations together in one household. Each person's role in the family is clearly defined. The father is the head of the family, and the mother stays home and takes care of the children. The children are secure in the home environment, cared for by the mother or another family member. Once in the United States, however, these roles suddenly change. The father may be unable to find employment and stay at home; the mother may work two jobs. The children may become translators for the parents.

When the children go to school, they may feel out of place because they "look different, dress oddly, and talk funny." They need moral support from their families. The parents may themselves feel lonely, homesick, depressed, isolated, and confused at this time, however. Consequently, because their own problems seem overwhelming, the parents are not equipped to deal with their children's problems and are unable to provide the support that the children need.

Liu and Yu (1975) noted that the Western view of the self and identity is different from the Oriental view. The Western view of self is individualistic and independent. In contrast, the Oriental sees the individual as part of the whole society in almost a selfless view. The Asian generally perceives the identity of self as part of the identity of the society. In the Chinese culture, there is a "big self," which refers to the society, and a "small self," which refers to the individual self. Because there is no small self without the big self, it is necessary to sacrifice oneself for one's country; individual autonomy is not valued as highly as the harmony of the society.

In terms of interpersonal communication, most Asians prefer to use "minimum message communication" (Gardner, 1983) rather than elaborations. The Asians rely very heavily on nonverbal cues in communication. Because nonverbal cues carry different meanings in different cultures, people from other cultures may misinterpret or misunderstand the Asians' messages, causing embarrassment and breakdowns in the communication process.

In spite of these numerous adjustment difficulties, many Asian immigrant children have adapted quickly to their new schools and have learned the English language well. For their parents, however, the struggle to modify their deeply rooted cultural and social habits often takes much longer.

Educational Adjustments and Conflicts

Philips (1983) studied the Warm Springs Indian children and found numerous and significant differences in the learning styles of the Indian children. Similarly, Trueba (1984) found a number of differences in the ways Mexican bilingual children participated in class. Wong-Fillmore (1984) investigated the language learning of Chinese immigrants and examined their learning styles and participant structure. Moulton (1984) discussed the differences of the classroom participation of students in China. All of these studies indicated that there is a wide range of preference in personal distance and degree of participation among the various cultural groups.

Most Asian children have been taught that they go to school to learn and that they must be obedient and respect the teachers. They generally use honorific terms to address their teachers and feel shy, uneasy, and uncomfortable when they talk to their teachers. In most Asian schools, students are told to be quiet during class and to remain in their assigned seats for the class. In Chinese schools, students must stand up and bow to the teacher to indicate respect and reverence when the teacher enters or leaves the classroom. The teacher's instructions are to be obeyed and never challenged. There is a definite social and psychological distance between the teacher and the students. These (unwritten) rules are to be followed without question.

With such an attitude, Asian children bow their head to the teacher, look down when talked to, giggle when embarrassed or reprimanded, and hand papers to the teacher with both hands. When praised, Asian students may feel uneasy and may not know how to respond appropriately. Their parents tell them that it is disrespectful to look someone in the eye, while their American teachers consider eye contact a sign of attention and respect. Teacher comments about poor eye contact and lack of responsiveness in Asian children may actually indicate a misunderstanding of Asian signs of respect.

Cultural conventions for class participation are clearly defined and obeyed by Asian schoolchildren. Asian children are often confused by the spontaneous and outspoken behaviors of their peers in American classrooms, viewing these behaviors as signs of disrespect for authority. Class participation and discussion may be foreign concepts to some of the Asian students, who often consider volunteering answers and information a bold and immodest practice. They may seem lost if they are asked to participate in the decision-making process regarding course content.

Asian parents revere teachers and expect them to assign a great deal of homework. Furthermore, the parents expect discipline in the classroom and may not approve of teachers who allow students a great deal of freedom. As a result, there are incongruencies between the parents' perception of the teachers' role and the teachers' own perception of their role. The conflicting messages given by teachers and parents confuse the children, sometimes leading to misbehavior. The children may be perceived as discipline problems, when they are, in fact, simply unfamiliar with the pragmatic and cultural-social rules of the school. Thus, it is imperative that educators understand the implications of the major cultural differences in learning style, teaching style, and participant structure. Most Asian children have been raised in a more rigid, disciplined and sheltered environment. They have learned to attend school with a formal attitude and should be helped to adjust to the relative informality and casual atmosphere of American schools.

In Asian countries, the educational process promotes passivity; students learn by listening, reading, observing, and imitating, rather than by engaging in critical thinking (Table 1-1). Students seldom ask questions in class, and teachers do not generally encourage students to ask questions. Teachers' questions are generally derived from their lectures and textbooks. Teachers are expected to lecture during class time; students, to take copious notes and memorize them. Examinations usually require students to recall factual information.

In the United States, teachers allow greater freedom in the classroom, encourage creativity, discussion, and debate. Students are expected to volunteer information and to ask questions. The shift from the lecture method of teaching to the freer learning environment, from memorization of facts to problem solving, from total dependence on teachers to self-reliance in finding information may

Table 1-1 Asian Attitudes toward Education

Asian Cultural Themes	Educational Implications
Education is a formal process.	Students are to engage in serious academic work. Teachers are to behave formally and are expected to lecture and provide information.
Teachers are to be highly respected.	Teachers are not to be interrupted. Students are reluctant to ask questions.
Humility is an important virtue.	Students are not to "show off" or volunteer information.
Reading of factual information is valuable study.	Reading of fiction is not considered serious study.
It is important for students to be orderly and obedient.	Students are to sit quietly and listen attentively.
Students learn by observation and by memorization.	Rote memory is an effective teaching tool.
Pattern practice and rote learning are "studying."	Homework in pattern practice is important and is expected.
Children must respect adults.	Children are expected to listen to adults.
Children must respect authority.	Teachers are not to be challenged or questioned.
Teachers have authority and control.	The class is run in an orderly manner and is highly controlled.
Rote learning is preferred over discovery learning. Teachers are carriers of knowledge and are transmitters of information.	Students do well in sheltered and structured activity—less peer interaction and group projects, more lectures and instruction.
Schooling is a serious process.	Students are expected to work in a quiet environment and are not to roam freely around the classroom.
Harmony is an important virtue.	Students avoid confrontation.
Filial piety is highly valued.	Children are obedient.

require a period of adjustment for the Asian language minority students. The prevailing Asian attitudes toward education present challenges for American educators and may affect the selection of strategies used to teach Asian students. Furthermore, the incongruencies between the expectations of American teachers and those of Asian parents must be considered in teaching Asian students (Table 1-2).

Table 1-2 Incongruencies between American Teachers' Expectations and Asian Parents' Expectations

American Teachers' Expectations	Asian Parents' Expectations
Students need to participate in classroom activities and discussion.	Students are to be quiet and obedient.
Students need to be creative.	Students should be told what to do.
Students learn through inquiries and debate.	Students learn through memorization and observation.
Asian students generally do well on their own.	Teachers need to teach; students need to "study."
Critical thinking is important. Analytical thinking is important.	It is important to deal with the real world.
Creativity and fantasy are to be encouraged.	Factual information is important; fantasy is not.
Problem solving is important.	Students should be taught the steps to solve problems.
Students need to ask questions.	Teachers are not to be challenged.
Reading is a way of discovering.	Reading is the decoding of information and facts.

Educational Styles

The Teachers

American teachers are friendly, open, and informal, whereas Asian teachers are reserved, serious, and formal. This discrepancy is difficult for the Asian students to accept, and teacher-student communication can break down as a result. In such cases, it is helpful for instructors to ask Asian students questions to determine whether the student has understood the concept or material presented. Because teachers and school personnel are accorded the highest respect, Asian students tend to maintain the "proper" social distance from teachers.

The Asian Parents

As noted previously, many Asian parents perceive a teacher who does not assign heavy homework loads as lenient and incompetent. They may also perceive the open classroom as uncontrolled, undisciplined, confusing, and unorganized. They value factual information and expect their children to learn facts.

Asian parents may view any request from school personnel for a conference as problematic. They often interpret such a request as an indication that their children are misbehaving at school and feel dismayed and ashamed. They may feel uncomfortable at such meetings, being unfamiliar not only with the concepts being discussed, but also with the entire social and linguistic milieu. In most cases, they prefer to leave educational decisions to the educators; therefore, they may appear unresponsive and unconcerned about the placement and curriculum of their children. In actuality, however, their reluctance to participate is a sign of respect, not apathy; they feel that they are not in a position to challenge the decisions and authority of school personnel.

The parents are also unfamiliar with the procedures required to develop an Individualized Education Program (IEP), finding the paperwork overwhelming and difficult to understand. Interpreters are often needed to facilitate communication and assure Asian parents that their children are not misbehaving, but simply need special education intervention.

Conclusion

Not all people from the same culture have the same values and beliefs; there are tremendous individual differences. For this reason, it is necessary to be extremely careful when making cultural assumptions. Nevertheless, an awareness of the general cultural and linguistic values of Asian minority populations is an essential tool for the speech-language-hearing specialist who provides services to these groups. Even though the clinician is unlikely to speak the native languages of these Asian minorities, an understanding of their cultural and linguistic values makes it possible for the clinician to communicate more effectively with them, to recognize many of their difficulties, to avoid potential conflicts, and to establish an atmosphere that will facilitate the provision of services.

CHAPTER 2

The Chinese

The word *China* is derived from the word *Tchina*, which first appeared during the Tsin Dynasty (255–202 B.C.). This name was then carried by Malay traders to India and other Western lands. In the classic writing of Europe, China is called Serica; its capital, Sera; and its people, Seres. In the name China xx, which literally means the Middle Kingdom, the word x indicates that the royal domain formed the center of the world and the realm of the nobles comprised the outer territories. The Chinese realm included five great divisions: (1) Han, (2) Manchuria, (3) Mongolia, (4) Chinese Turkestan, and (5) Tibet (Figure 2-1).

Geographically, China is situated to the north of Indochina and to the south of the Soviet Union. A country rich in history and culture, China has influenced all the Asian cultures. The population is composed of various ethnic groups, including the Han, Mongolian, Tibetan, and Manchurian tribes. There are more than 1.2 billion Chinese, representing one-quarter of the world's population. The Han group is by far the largest group in China, as it is more than 90% of the total population. The remainder of the population consists of more than 55 minority peoples, who inhabit more than one-half of the country's territory. Different from the Han group in language, customs, historical development, religion, and race, these ethnic groups include

- South: The Mias (Hmong) people are dispersed throughout Southern China, Vietnam, Laos, and Thailand. They vary in dialect and styles of farming. They settled in distant mountains. The Li are natives of Hainan Island.
- Southeast: The main groups are the Tujia, She, and Yao. Kaoshan is the term applied to the aboriginal mountain peoples of Taiwan. Their languages stem from the Malayo-Polynesian group.
- Northeast: The main group is the Manchu. They hunt, breed deer, tend flocks, and farm. The Koreans also filtered into this region.
- North Central: The main group is the Mongol people, who are seminomadic and follow their flocks in summer. The Hui are Muslim and are represented in many occupations.
- Southwest: The Zhuang are the largest of the minorities and share with the Dai (ethnic Thailand) linguistic roots and a love of singing and dancing. Another

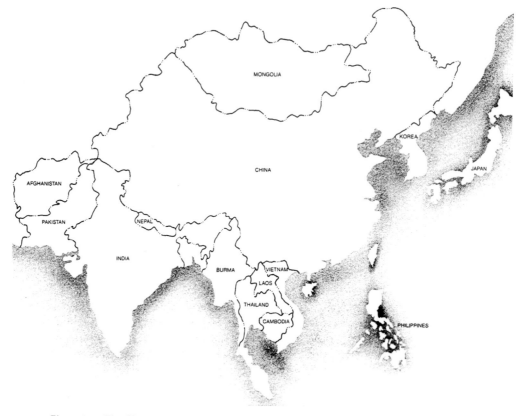

Figure 2-1 The Chinese Realm

---

group is the Yao; they raise rice, maize, and sweet potatoes. The Yi people are warriors and have evolved into an aristocratic society with a religion based on the reading of sacred writing.

- Tibetan highlands: The Tibetans inhabit a high, desolate region surrounded by mountains. They herd yaks, sheep, and goats, and they farm peas, barley, and tubers.
- Xinjiang: The Kazak and Kirgiz are herders of sheep and goats. They now live in communes in the winter.

These diverse peoples produce most of China's livestock and have in their territories most of China's mineral resources.

Historical Background

Chinese history dates back 5,000 years. The three main dynasties were Han, Yuen, and Chin. It was during the Han Dynasty (206 B.C. to 220 A.D.) that China expanded into Central Asia and Mongolia. Traders traveled on the Silk Road as far as Rome. The Mongols overturned the Han majority and ruled China during the Yuen Dynasty under their khans (1260–1368). Later, the Manchurians ruled China as the last dynasty (Chin Dynasty, 1644–1911).

Dr. Sun Yat-Sen and his followers overthrew the Chin Dynasty in 1911 and founded the Republic of China. In 1938, Japan invaded China; the resultant Sino-

Japanese War lasted 8 years, until the end of World War II. After the War, the Communist and the Nationalist Chinese struggled in civil war until 1949, when the Communist Chinese were victorious and founded the People's Republic of China. After the Communist revolution, comprehensive policies on regional autonomy, training programs, and the development of native languages were issued for minorities.

The Kuomingtung (Nationalist Chinese) went to the island of Taiwan, situated in the South China Sea 100 miles off the shore of China. In 1590, the Portuguese had sailed through the South China Sea and exclaimed, "isla formosa!" (beautiful island) at the sight of the island; for this reason, Taiwan is sometimes called Formosa. The first group of Chinese sailed to the island in 230 A.D. More Chinese moved to the island during the Suey Dynasty (581–600 A.D.). During the Yuen Dynasty, Taiwan officially became part of China. During the Ming Dynasty (1522–1635 A.D.), sea pirates occupied much of the island. The Dutch landed at Tainan, a southern seaport, in 1626 and ruled Taiwan for 38 years, but they were driven out by General Cheng-Kung Cheng. Taiwan was under Chinese rule until the end of the First Sino-Japanese War, when it was ceded to Japan (1893). Taiwan was then under Japanese rule until 1945, when it was returned to China. Under Japanese rule, the Japanese language was Taiwan's official language.

Hong Kong (Victoria) is situated northwest of Taiwan. It was under Chinese rule until the end of the first Opium War (1839), after which it was ceded to England. Kowloon, across Hong Kong harbor, was ceded to England after the second Opium War (1856). Both Hong Kong and Kowloon will be returned to China in 1997.

Ethnic Chinese

Chinese have been settling in all parts of Southeast Asia for centuries. Between 1860 and 1930, many Chinese from Canton (Kuangtong) and Fukien (Fujian) moved to Southeast Asia for economic reasons. Because of governmental pressure, many were forced to change their names and adopt the outward cultural characteristics of their country of residence. These ethnic Chinese continued to perceive themselves as Chinese, however, and tried to retain their own language and culture as well. Even today, there are Chinese in all Southeast Asian countries.

During the French colonial period, the ethnic Chinese in Indochina established Chinese schools, using Mandarin as the language of instruction. Many went to the schools of their host country during the day and to Chinese school at night and during the weekend. During the 1940s and 1950s, the development of nationalism in Vietnam, Laos, and Cambodia made it difficult for the Chinese schools to survive, as these schools were believed to inhibit Chinese assimilation. Fearing persecution, a large number of ethnic Chinese refugees left Vietnam, Laos, and Cambodia. The ethnic Chinese who have fled Indochina as refugees may speak a Chinese dialect (e.g., Mandarin, Hakka, Cantonese, Min, or Chaocho [Chiu Jew]). They also speak Vietnamese, Laotian, or Cambodian, depending on their country of residence.

Chinese Traditions and Values

The notion of family in China is a comprehensive one. Each member of the family has a role and a position that are clearly defined through an intricate kinship system. For example, an older brother is called a 哥, a younger brother is called a 弟, an older sister is called a 姊 , a younger sister is called a 妹 , an older male cousin from the father's side is called a 堂哥 a younger female cousin from the mother's side is called a 表妹, and a younger male cousin from the father's side is called 堂弟. Furthermore, the mother's younger sister is 姨 , the father's younger brother is 叔 , the mother's older brother is 舅 , and the father's younger sister is 姑. A married woman calls her father-in-law 公 and her mother-in-law 婆 , while her husband calls his father-in-law 岳父 and his mother-in-law 岳母. Thus, kinship terms make it easy to determine precise relationships. Kinship terms also serve as a reminder of the specific roles and duties of family members. Children are taught while very young to call relatives by the proper terms and are not allowed to address people by their first name.

The Chinese culture places a heavy emphasis on the strength of the family as a large unit and the importance of respect for elders in the family. Grandparents are accorded the highest respect and authority. Members of the extended family, such as uncles and aunts, are given equal respect and may reside in the same household. A family member who is not married usually stays with a member of his or her family. The new policy on zero population growth in the People's Republic of China will have a significant impact on the future of the family structure.

According to Chinese history, Confucius remained by the tomb of his mother for many years after her death to show his filial piety. Such virtue is highly regarded by the Chinese. Traditional Chinese parents will sacrifice personal needs to provide for their children, but in return expect unquestioning obedience from their children. Children are considered "good" only if they do what their parents want them to do. Moreover, children are expected to take care of their parents in their old age.

The hierarchy within a traditional Chinese family is well defined. The father is responsible for all family members. The mother is responsible for the care of the children; if there are problems with the children, the mother is blamed for her lack of attention. The oldest son must be obedient to his parents and is responsible for the care of his younger siblings. He is also expected to make sacrifices for the sake of the younger siblings. The daughter defers to her parents and older brother. She also has responsibility for the routine care of her younger siblings, including bathing, dressing, changing, feeding, and sometimes, cooking. The younger children are to obey their parents and older siblings.

Young Chinese children are nurtured and made to feel very secure in their home environment. During the early childhood years, young children are generally cared for by family members. They typically wear more clothing than necessary, because their parents and grandparents do not want them to get cold. Someone feeds them until they are 4 years of age, because parents are concerned that their children may not eat enough if they feed themselves. They are not encouraged to go outside to play, as they may get dirty. Perceiving young children as helpless, parents tend to be more permissive with them. Even so, discipline is an important part of the Chinese culture. Parents use shaming, withdrawal of love, and the implication of "loss of face" when disciplining their children. They constantly remind their children that any misbehavior reflects on the entire family. Physical punishment is also viewed differently as well as motivational style.

Parents teach their children to behave according to strict rules. They expect their children to follow the example of their older siblings. Parents generally take their young children to family gatherings and social occasions, such as weddings, dinner parties, and festivals, where they listen to adult conversation and watch adult behavior. Thus, Chinese children learn by observation and imitation from a very young age.

One of the most important ideals of the Chinese culture is the pursuit and maintenance of harmony. Children are told not to be aggressive nor to seek confrontation, but rather to try to maintain harmony. Value is placed on an outward calmness and on control of such undesirable emotions as anger, jealousy, hostility, aggression, and self-pity.

Almost all traditional Chinese families expect their children to do well in school and to go into a particular field, such as research, science, medicine, or business. Children are taught to believe that the only way to succeed in life is to work hard and respect authority. Such views may be inconsistent with the Western philosophy of the balance of work and play. Many Chinese consider individual recreation wasteful and self-indulgent; they do not have hobbies and do not understand the importance that Americans place on individual hobbies and interests. Very few Chinese are athletes in comparison to the multitude of the Chinese population.

If a family member is successful, the entire family receives credit. Traditional Chinese families tend to be modest about individual achievement and seldom talk about such accomplishments, however. Expressions of pride are considered arrogant and in conflict with the ideals of humility. While families may be very proud of their children's achievements, they may still minimize these achievements in public to show their sense of humility and modesty. Furthermore, parents do not praise their children readily, even when they excel in school, since such excellence is expected. If a child does poorly in school or needs special attention, the parents often feel ashamed, perceiving the child's difficulties as a sign of their own failure and, therefore, as a loss of face.

Parents take their children to Chinese schools on weekends and expect them to learn Chinese and to maintain the culture. Such dual expectations often create conflicts, causing children to rebel and to resent the Chinese language and the culture. As a result, a large number of American-born Chinese do not speak the Chinese language.

Traditionally, teachers are highly respected. The Cultural Revolution in China (1964–1974) was an exception to this rule, however. The 10-year cultural revolution did great damage to educational institutions, research efforts, and individual scholars. Educational facilities were damaged; public monuments defaced; teachers and scholars publicly humiliated and imprisoned; books, art work, and important documents destroyed; and schools closed. In the last decade, much of the ground lost has been regained, and teachers in China are accorded great respect in present day China.

Some Chinese believe in the horoscope. Depending on the time of birth according to the lunar calendar, a person is born in a year named for one of 12 animals in a 12-year astrological cycle: rat, ox, tiger, rabbit, dragon, serpent, horse, ram, monkey, rooster, dog, and pig. It is not unusual for a Chinese to ask about another's age or birth sign. Many parents name their children according to the year of their birth or the place of their birth. For example, some children are named little dragon, little tiger, born in Hunan, or born in Taiwan.

Chinese Immigration into the United States

Early Chinese Immigration

The Chinese first emigrated to the United States almost two centuries ago. The documentation of their early history is not extensive; the information available is drawn primarily from personal life histories, contemporary news reports, government documents, and family anecdotes passed from generation to generation.

The first records showing the arrival of Chinese in the United States date from 1785, when three seamen from China landed in Baltimore. The first Chinese contract laborers (coolies) arrived in 1845. Chinese started to come in greater numbers after 1848, the year in which gold was discovered near Coloma, California. The news about the "mountains of gold" reached China, and 20,000 Chinese went to San Francisco (translated "old gold mountain" in Chinese) to prospect for gold.

By 1870, one-third of the miners in California were Chinese. The enactment of discriminatory laws, such as the California Foreign Miner's Tax, failed to discourage the Chinese miners. They worked for meager wages in abandoned mines until claims were exhausted. At approximately the same time, thousands of Chinese were hired to build the railroads. Many were killed while completing hazardous tasks with explosives. The railroad between the West and the East was finished in 1869, after which the Chinese continued to build rail links throughout California. In addition to working in the mines and on the railroads, Chinese immigrants worked in the farming industry. In the late 1890s, there was a strong anti-Chinese movement, and the Japanese began to replace the Chinese as laborers in the farming industry.

The first Chinese Exclusion Act, passed by the U.S. Congress in 1882, banned the entrance of Chinese laborers for 10 years. In 1906, the San Francisco Board of Education ordered that all Chinese, Japanese, and Korean children be segregated in an Oriental School. In 1924, the U.S. Congress passed another exclusion act, prohibiting the entrance of Chinese women into the United States. In 1943, President Franklin Roosevelt abolished all immigration rules against the Chinese and set a quota of 105 Chinese immigrants per year. The quota has since been increased many times.

Recent Chinese Immigration

Since World War II, Chinese have been coming to the United States from Taiwan and Hong Kong. Most have come primarily to study or to join their families. In recent years, however, more Chinese immigrants have come to the United States for business purposes. Many Chinese from Hong Kong have come to the United States because they fear the consequences of the Communist takeover of Hong Kong in 1997. Since President Richard Nixon's ping-pong diplomacy, many Chinese from the People's Republic of China have applied for immigration to the United States in order to join their family members, or to study. It is estimated that there are 10,000 students from China in American institutions of higher learning.

Not only do recent Chinese immigrants have a variety of motivations and backgrounds, but also they speak a diverse group of languages. Therefore, the following discussion is limited to some general features of the Han language and the two most common dialects, Mandarin and Cantonese.

Chinese Language Considerations

The languages spoken by the peoples of China are classified into five broad language groupings: (1) Sino-Tibetan, (2) Altaic, (3) Malayo-Polynesian, (4) Austro-Asiatic, and (5) Indo-European. More than 80 languages and hundreds of dialects are spoken in China. Some of them are closely related; others are mutually unintelligible. Han belongs to the Sino-Tibetan group. Of the Chinese population, 94% are reported to speak Han 漢 and its dialects: Mandarin, Wu, Yue, (Cantonese) Xiang, Gan, Kejia, and Min.

More than two-thirds of the Chinese population speak Mandarin dialects. Although Han dialects differ greatly in their phonetic and tonal aspects, they share the same written system. The government of the People's Republic of China has simplified the traditional written system and developed the Pinyin system, which is based on the Roman alphabet.

The Chinese dialects are extremely complex. The term *dialect* is used to describe two mutually auditorily incomprehensible systems. For example, the word *sit* 坐 is pronounced

tsuo in Mandarin
suo in Cantonese
zei in Taiwanese

Speakers of two different Chinese dialects cannot understand each other, even though their words are graphically represented by the same character.

Chinese is a tone language. Each character is phonetically represented by a single syllable. There are many two-character words, for example, airplane fēchī. Each syllable has its tone mark. Each Han dialect has its own tonal system. In Mandarin Chinese, there are four tones (and a neutral tone). For example, the Mandarin syllable *ma* can be represented by the following:

1st tone	High level	mā	媽	mother
2nd tone	Rising	má	麻	hemp
			什麼	what
			痳痺	paralysis
3rd tone	Falling-rising	mǎ	馬	horse
			瑪瑙	agate
			螞蟻	ant
			碼	yard
			榪	clamp
4th tone	Falling	mǎ	罵	to scold

The same spoken syllable has different meanings, depending on the tone and the various characters that the syllable represents. For example,

1st tone shī	2nd tone shí	3rd tone shǐ	4th tone shì
師 teacher	時 time	史 history	士 scholar
獅 lion	蒔 to plant	使 employ	仕 fill an office
濕 wet	食 to eat	駛 to sail	侍 serve
詩 poetry	拾 to pick up	始 to begin	恃 depend
噬 bite	十 ten	纚 long	氏 family
豕 pig	石 stone	矢 dart	舐 lick
弛 relax	蝕 eclipse	匙 spoon	事 affair
施 bestow	碩 great		世 an age

Chinese Dialects Spoken in the United States

The two main dialects spoken by the Chinese in the United States are Cantonese and Mandarin. The majority of early Chinese immigrants had been from Cantonese-speaking 廣東 regions, such as Hor.g Kong and the Province of Canton. Among them, some speak Taishanese 台山, a subdialect of the Canton Province. Many Vietnamese refugees are of Chinese descent and speak Cantonese. Similarly, many Chinese families from other Asian countries (e.g., Singapore, Malaysia, and the Philippines), speak Cantonese, Min, and Hakka (Kejia). Cantonese is spoken in Chinatowns across the United States.

The second most common dialect spoken by Chinese immigrants in the United States is Mandarin, spoken by immigrants from Taiwan and Mainland China. Their language includes the Peking (Beijing) dialect pronunciation and the grammar of Mandarin.

Chinese Written System

Chinese characters are sometimes called ideographs or logographs (Exhibit 2-1). The graphic form of the characters has gone through many evolutionary

Exhibit 2-1 Chinese Ideographs

日	sun	二	two
月	moon	三	three
人	man	川	river
大	woman	凹	concave
田	field	凸	convex
木	wood	上	up
林	forest	下	down
森	woods	中	middle
一	one	大	big
		小	little

changes (Figure 2-2). The variations evolved from the pictographs carved on oracle bone of almost 4,000 years ago, Chuan of Chin Dynasty (221–2007 B.C.), and Li of Han Dynasty to the cursive Kai calligraphy of modern times (Table 2-1). The forming of the characters has also gone through evolutionary changes, and Table 2-1 demonstrates this point well. The evolution of the written language is seen in characters from sun, moon, mouth, water, etc.

Both the Korean and the Japanese languages have borrowed from the Chinese written system. The Japanese words that have a Chinese origin are called Kanji 漢字 which means Han characters. Unlike the English-speaking peoples, who create new words for new things, the Chinese compose new words by combining two characters or particles. For example, the character 車 means vehicle and is combined with the following characters to mean a variety of vehicles:

train	火車	trailer	拖車
cable car	電車	truck	卡車
automobile	汽車	station wagon	旅行車
bicycle	自行車	bus	公共汽車
cart	手拉車	buggy	馬車
motorcycle	機車		

Each character has a prescribed sequence of strokes, and they are learned by continuous practice and visual memorization. Schoolchildren in Taiwan are ex-

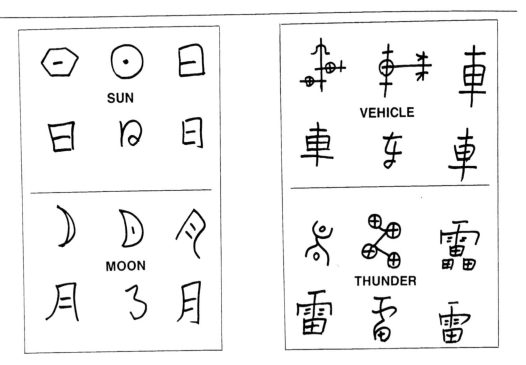

Figure 2-2 Evolution of the Chinese Written Language

Table 2-1 Chinese Characters: From Ancient to Modern Times

Ancient Form	Modern Form	Pronounced	Meaning
⊙	日	rì	Sun or day
☽	月	yuè	Moon or month
酉	酒	jiǔ	Wine
⋀⋀	山	shān	Mountain
田	田	tián	Field
▽	口	kǒu	Mouth
⫲⫲	水	shuǐ	Water
⫲⫲	川	chuān	River
⼥	女	nǚ	Woman
⼿	手	shǒu	Hand
⊖	回	huí	Return to

Source: From *Speaking of Chinese* (p. 15) by R. Chang and M.S. Chang, 1978, New York, NY: W. W. Norton & Company, Inc. Copyright 1978 by W. W. Norton & Company, Inc. Reprinted by permission.

pected to learn this written system and the national phonetic system. The children in China are taught the simplified version of the written language 簡字 and the Pinyin system of pronunciation.

Phonology of Mandarin and Cantonese

A syllable in Mandarin or Cantonese consists of segmental and suprasegmental features (Figure 2-3). Segmental features include an initial consonant (optional) and a final sound (Tables 2-2 through 2-6). Suprasegmental features include the distinct tones that are an intrinsic part of the phonological makeup of a Chinese syllable. The Mandarin tone system is presented in Table 2-7.

Tone				
	Final			
		Rime		
				Ending
Initial	Medial	Nucleus	Vocalic ending	Consonantal ending

Figure 2-3 Syllable Structure of Mandarin and Cantonese

Source: From *Drills and Exercises in Mandarin Pronunciation* by T.M. Yeh, 1982, Taipei: National Taiwan University.

Table 2-2 Mandarin Initial Consonants

Manner of Articulation			Bilabial — Upper Lip (Lower lip)	Labio-dental — Upper Teeth	Apico-dental — Lower Teeth (Tongue tip)	Alveolar — Alveolar Ridge (Tongue tip)	Apico-palatal — Hard Palate (Tongue tip)	Lamino-palatal — Hard Palate (Tongue blade)	Dorso-velar — Velor (Dorsum)
STOPS	Voiceless	Unasp.	p			t			k
STOPS	Voiceless	Asp.	p‘			t‘			k‘
AFFRICATES	Voiceless	Unasp.			ts		tʂ	tɕ	
AFFRICATES	Voiceless	Asp.			ts‘		tʂ‘	tɕ‘	
NASALS	Voiced		m			n			(ŋ)
LATERAL	Voiced					l			
SPIRANTS	Voiceless			f	s		ʂ	ɕ	x
SPIRANTS	Voiced						ʐ		

*Occurs in the final position of a syllable only
Unasp.: Unaspiration
Asp.: Aspiration

Table 2-3 Cantonese Initial Sounds

p′	(aspirated)	p
p	(unaspirated)	b
t′		t
t		d
k′		k
k		g
t′	(aspirated)	ch
t	(unaspirated)	j
K′w	(aspirated)	kw
kw	(unaspirated)	gw
m		m
n		n
n		ng
f		f
l		l
h		h
		s
j		y
w		w

Source: From Assessment of Chinese Speaking Limited English Proficient Students with Special Needs, by Special Education Resource Network, 1986, Sacramento: California State Department of Education.

Table 2-4 Cantonese Consonants in the Yale Romanization System

b	p	m	f
d	t	n	l
j	ch	s	h
g	k	ng	y
gw	kw	w	

Source: From *Assessment of Chinese Speaking Limited English Proficient Students with Special Needs,* by Special Education Resource Network, 1986, Sacramento: California State Department of Education.

Table 2-5 Cantonese Vowels in the Yale Romanization System

a	aa	e	eu	i	o	u	yu
aai	ai	ei	eui		oi	ui	
aau	au			iu	ou		
aam	am			im			
aan	an		eun	in	on	un	yun
aang	ang	eng	eung	ing	ong	ung	
aap	ap		eut	ip			
aat	at	ek	euk	it	ot	ut	yut
aak	ak			ik	ok	uk	

Source: From *Assessment of Chinese Speaking Limited English Proficient Students with Special Needs,* by Special Education Resource Network, 1986, Sacramento: California State Department of Education.

Table 2-6 Mandarin Final Sounds Table

	a	o		ai	ei	au	ou	an	n	a	
i	ia		ie			iau	iou	ian	in	ia	i
u	ua	uo		uai	uei			uan	un	ua	u
y			ye					yan	un	uy	

Source: From *Drills and Exercises in Mandarin Pronunciation,* by T.M. Yeh, 1982, Taipei: National Taiwan University.

The number of Cantonese tones is still debated. The Yale Romanization System recognizes seven tones in Cantonese (Boyle, 1970; Table 2-8). Some linguists argue that there are nine tones in Cantonese, however (Table 2-9).

Certain tones change in tone category when they are in particular sequences; such a phenomenon is called ''tone sandhi.'' When two Mandarin third tones appear consecutively in an utterance, for example, the first third tone becomes a second tone. Thus, the phrase *good horse* in Mandarin is produced as

hau 好 ma 馬 (good horse)

好 good (hǎu) is a third tone, 馬 horse (mǎ) is also a third tone. When the two words are combined to mean good horse, the hǎu becomes hau.

English vs. Chinese (Mandarin and Cantonese)

A comparative analysis of the phonetic systems of English and Chinese reveals the features of English that are most likely to cause difficulty for Chinese speak-

Table 2-7 The Tones in Mandarin

	Pitch Level	Duration and Direction
First tone	High Half-high Mid Half-low Low	
Second tone	High Half-high Mid Half-low Low	
Third tone	High Half-high Mid Half-low Low	
Fourth tone	High Half-high Mid Half-low Low	

ers who are learning English. For example, English has consonant blends that can occur in different positions:

1. double blends
   a. initial position: *spy, bribe, clown*
   b. final position: *ask gasp*
   c. medial position: *basket, mustard*
2. triple blends
   a. initial position: *splash, spring*
   b. final position: *asks, lisps*

There are no consonant blends in Mandarin or Cantonese, however, and Chinese learners may find the English blends a "mouthful."

Because Chinese characters are each composed of a single syllable, the rules for syllabification and syllabic stress in English may present difficulty for a

Table 2-8 Seven Tones of Cantonese

Tone	Sound	Chinese Character	Meaning
High-level	sī	詩	Poem
High-falling	sī	思	To think
High-rising	si	史	History
Mid-level	si	試	To try
Low-falling	sīh	時	Time
Low-rising	sih	市	City
Low-level	sih	事	Event

Source: From *Assessment of Chinese Speaking Limited English Proficient Students with Special Needs*, by Special Education Resource Network, 1986, Sacramento: California State Department of Education.

Table 2-9 The Cantonese Tone System

Traditional Tone Class	Tone Values	Status (Etic or Emic)	Examples
Upper even	55	Emic	/fan/'grade'
	54 (53)	Etic (unconditioned free variant of 55)	
Upper rising	25	Emic	/fan/'powder'
Upper going	33	Emic	/fan/'sleep'
Lower even	11	Emic	/fan/'burn'
Lower rising	13	Emic	/fan/'strive'
Lower going	22	Emic	/fan/'share'
High entering	5	Etic	/fan/'sudden'
Mid entering	3	Etic	/fat/'law'
Low entering	2	Etic	/fat/'punish'

Etic = difference in meaning
Emic = no difference in meaning
Source: From *Assessment of Chinese Speaking Limited English Proficient Students with Special Needs,* by Special Education Resource Network, 1986, Sacramento: California State Department of Education.

Mandarin or Cantonese speaker. These speakers may sound telegraphic and may truncate English words.

In Mandarin, there are two finals, the sonorants, namely, /n/ and /ŋ/; in Cantonese, there are seven finals: /m/, /n/, /ŋ/ and /p/, /t/, /k/, and /ʔ/. In English, however, there are many finals: /p/, /m/, /n/, /b/, /g/, /k/, /f/, /d/, /z/, /t/, /ʃ/, /tʒ/, /l/, /r/, /dʒ/, /ʒ/, /v/, /s/, /θ/, and /ð/. Finding it difficult to produce the final consonants in English words, Chinese speakers learning English may sometimes omit them, for example, *offi* for *office,* *fi* for *fish,* *cat* for *cats.*

Chinese learners may use Chinese sounds when speaking English when those sounds are phonetically similar in the two languages. For example, Mandarin speakers frequently produce the English phoneme /tʃ/ in *chair* as /tɕ/; Cantonese speakers frequently produce the English phoneme /ʃ/ in *social* as /s/. These speakers may also substitute a Chinese sound for an English sound that does not exist in Chinese. For example, they may use *sin* for *thin,* as there is no such sound as /θ/ in either Mandarin or Cantonese. After more than a decade of study, linguists have concluded that these difficulties arise in part from the fact that sounds are perceived and produced in functional categories (Ojemann & Whitaker, 1978; Sasanuma, 1974; Tzeng & Wang, 1971; Wang, 1976). Thus, the phonetic system of one language interferes with the learning process when those who speak that language are trying to learn another (Tables 2-10 and 2-11).

The vowel system of Cantonese may also interfere with the efforts of the Cantonese speaker to learn to speak English correctly (Table 2-12). For example, Cantonese speakers may substitute

e for ɛ and æ	snake / snack
	raid / red
i for I	eat / it
o for ɔ	boat / bought
	sew / saw
u for ʊ	roof / rough
or	
a for ʌ	got / gut

Table 2-10 Possible Phonetic Interferences of Mandarin in Learning English

Interference	Sound	Position	Example
Substitution	s/θ	Initial	sum/thumb
		Medial	Kassy/Kathy
	f/θ	Final	baf/bath
	s/θ	Final	bas/bath
	d/ð	Initial	dis/this
		Medial	broder/brother
		Medial	someding/something
	z/ð	Initial	zis/this
		Medial	brozer/brother
		Medial	closing/clothing
	f/v	Initial	fine/vine
		Initial	fase/vase
		Medial	surface/service
	w/v	Initial	wery/very
		Medial	surwase/service
Confusion	r/l	Initial	right/light
		Blend	crown/clown
	l/r	Initial	lice/rice
		Initial	light/right
Omission	/s/	Final	gra/grace
	/z/	Final	ma/maze
	/f/	Final	wi/wife
	/v/	Final	fi/five
	/k/	Final	ca/cake
	/p/	Final	kee/keep
	/g/	Final	ba/bag
	/t/	Final	boo/boot
	/d/	Final	be/bed
	/ʃ/	Final	fi/fish
	/tʃ/	Final	cat/catch
	/l/	Final	ba/ball
	/r/	Final	ca/car
	/θ/	Final	wrea/wreath
	/ə/	Final	wrea/wreathe
Addition	əin blends		belue/blue
			gooda/good
			morninga/morning
			picnica/picnic
			sapaghetti/spaghetti
Approximation			tçair/chair
			çee/see
			tçtç/judge
Shortening or lengthening the vowels			seat/sit
			heat/hit
			sit/seat
			it/eat

Chinese speakers frequently misplace English word stress, for example, tele-'vision or sepa'rately. Moreover, the intonational patterns of the English language differ from those of Mandarin and Cantonese. Because intonation patterns differentiate important meanings (e.g., statements from questions, demands from requests, excitement from sarcasm, enthusiasm from indiffer-

Table 2-11 Possible Phonetic Interferences of Cantonese in Learning English

Interference	Sound	Position	Example
Substitution	s/θ	Initial	sorn/thorn
	f/θ	Final	wif/with
	d/ð	Initial	dis/this
		Medial	broder/brother
	s/z	Initial	sue/zoo
		Final	mase/maze
		Medial, final	scizzorz/scissors
	f/v	Initial	fine/vine
		Medial	wafy/wavy
		Medial	wafe/wave
	w/v	Initial	wery/very
		Medial	heawy/heavy
	l/r	Initial	light/right
		Medial	Maly/Mary
		Final	cal/car
	w/wʌ	Initial	wear/where
	s/sh	Initial	sue/shoe
		Medial	soso/social
		Final	was/wash
	z/zdʒ	Initial	zuce/juice
Omission	/s/	Final	dre/dress
	/z/	Final	free/freeze
	/f/	Final	bee/beef
	/v/	Final	hi/hive
	/b/	Final	Bo/Bob
	/d/	Final	Te/Ted
	/g/	Final	mu/mug
	/tʃ/	Final	mat/match
	/ʃ/	Final	wa/wash
	/l/	Final	ba/ball
	/r/	Final	ca/car
	/ts/	Final	ba/bats
	/ð/	Final	brea/breathe

Table 2-12 Comparison of English and Cantonese Vowel Systems

		Vowels	Diphthongs/Triphthongs	
English	ɑ	father	ai	aisle
	e	make	au	now
	æ	sat	ɔi	coil
	I	fatigue		
	ε	red		
	ɪ	it		
	o	hope		
	ɔ	sauce		
	ð	fur		
		never		
	u	true		
	ʋ	put		
	ʌ	under		
	ə	about		
Cantonese	a		aa, aai, ai	
	e		ei, eu, eui	
	i		aau, au, ai, i, iu ou	
	o			
	u			

ence), it is crucial for both the speaker and the listener to understand these distinctions. It may be difficult for Chinese speakers to learn the overall intonation patterns of the English language, however, which creates problems in communication. Morphological and syntactical difficulties compound these communication problems (Table 2-13).

Several *semantic* problems arise for the Chinese speaker learning English. The same meaning may be expressed by very different words; for example, the literal translation for the expression *turn on the light* in English is open the light in Chinese. A single English word may have a number of meanings, and each is understood in its context; direct translation may be misleading and inappropriate. The sign *Do Not Pass* may discourage a Chinese driver from continuing because the word *pass* in Chinese may mean *go through here*. Words have their own connotations; the word *cat* in the expression *fat cat* does not mean a *cat*, for example. The word *foxy* applied to a person means a whole set of characteristics unknown to a Chinese learning English. Such connotations are culturally loaded and must be learned in context through experience. Colloquial expressions, such as *you bet, no sweat,* and *I see,* can be extremely difficult for Chinese to understand and may lead to confusion. In English, see, look, read, and watch are used in different contexts, whereas, in Chinese, one word is used for all four meanings. Chinese may experience difficulty in selecting the correct word for the right context.

Pragmatic Differences between English and Chinese

The pragmatic rules of the Chinese language differ a great deal from those of the English language:

- turn taking. Chinese generally do not ask questions or interrupt during a lecture. Students may appear passive and nonparticipatory.
- greeting. Chinese may ask "Have you eaten?" when greeting another person; the socially correct response is "Yes." Similarly, the correct response for the American greeting, "How are you?" is "Fine," whether it is true or not.
- social distance. Children are told to respect teachers and to maintain a proper social distance from them. Because social distance is judged by such attributes as age, status, marital status, Chinese consider the following questions appropriate:
  - How old are you? ("What is your honorable age?")
  - Where do you work? ("Where is your esteemed office?")
  - Are you married?
  These questions may be considered rude by an American, however.

- kinship terms. Chinese seem to be more precise in depicting human relationships, and English tends to be more precise in the field of quantitative sciences. Chinese speakers learning English may seek counterparts of kinship terms in English and may have difficulty adopting the American system. They may ask, "What do you mean? Is he your younger sister's husband or your husband's older brother?"
- proximity. Chinese do not generally hug or kiss, or express their emotions in public. Girls hold hands and dance with one another, although boys generally do not.

Table 2-13   Common Morphological and Syntactical Errors of Chinese Speakers Learning English

	Error	Example
Plural markers	Omissions	I see two girl.
		I see two mouse.
	Overregularization	I see two sheeps.
Copula	Omission	I _____ going to school now.
		She _____ making noise.
	Lack of inflection	I is going.
	Double marking	Is this is a pencil sharpener?
Auxiliary do	Omission	He _____ not want go.
	Lack of inflection	He do not have money.
Verb have	Lack of inflection	He have no time.
	Omission	You _____ been there.
Past tense markers	Omission	He go yesterday.
		He want come last week.
		I eat cake.
	Overregularization	I eated a cake.
		He sented me a book.
	Double marking	She didn't went home.
Interrogative	Misordering	You are there?
	Omission of morpheme	You like this?
Perfect auxiliary	Omission	I have eat _____.
		He have eat _____.
	Overgeneralization	He had wented.
Subjunctive		If he come, I will talk to him.
Singular present tense	Lack of inflection	She go to school.
	Addition of grammatical morpheme	You goes there.
Article	Omission	I see _____ dog.
		She read _____ book.
	Overgeneralization	She went the home.
Preposition	Misuse	I am in home./I am at home.
	Omission	I am going _____ Los Angeles./I am going to Los Angeles.
Pronouns	Overuse	Him is here.
		Him and I are here.
	Confusion in substitution	He said that./She said that.
		He said his husband will come./She said her husband will come.
Demonstratives	Overuse	I want that books.
Possessive	Omission	I go my mom _____ house.
	Misuse	This him book./This is his book.
Conjunction	Omission	I don't know _____ he come not come.
		You _____ I good friends. (You and I are good friends).
Comparative	Wrong use	This cake is gooder than that cake.
	Double marking	This is more bigger than that.
Negation	Double marking	I don't have no more.
	Omission	I no have _____.
Subject-verb-object relationship	Misordering	I wrote out it.
		I picked up it.
	Omission	I like./I like it.

- paralinguistic rules. Chinese often attempt to keep their faces expressionless. Although young children may stare at a stranger, staring at people is generally considered impolite. "Ladies," supposed to be more reserved, generally look downward and appear to be "shy." As a result, Chinese tend not to maintain "good" eye contact, which may be perceived unfavorably by Westerners. A giggle is a sign of embarrassment; a Chinese who is reprimanded may giggle rather than respond to the accusation. Gestures are often used to convey meaning, but the same gestures may mean very different things to Chinese and to Americans.
- politeness. Chinese are taught to be humble, and when praised, are generally embarrassed. When someone says "thank you," the correct response is generally "No need to thank me."

Conclusion

Clearly, a knowledge of the cultural and pragmatic characteristics of Chinese speakers is essential to successful interaction and communication with the Chinese students who have limited English proficiency (LEP), since these children bring to school very different communication skills. In order to determine whether Chinese LEP students have a language disorder, clinicians must work with interpreters to gather information about the students' competence in their native language. Clinicians must remember that linguistic interferences and differences are *not* deviancies. Research on the acquisition of a second language can be helpful in providing an appropriate assessment for Chinese LEP students and laying a good foundation for further diagnostic work-up and intervention.

CHAPTER 3

The Indochinese:
The Vietnamese, Laotians, Hmong, and Cambodians

Indochina is geographically situated on a peninsula to the south of China and to the east of India. It comprises Vietnam, Thailand, Laos, Cambodia, and Burma (Figure 3-1). Because there are plenty of fish in the rivers and the land is fertile, the region is often referred to as the "land of fish and rice." The weather is warm, and rainfall is sufficient for farming. These countries have similar foods, geography, and climate; there are some dissimilarities in culture, way of life, and religions, however. Since there are very few Thais and Burmese in the United States and most people refer to the Indochinese as Vietnamese, Laotians, and Cambodians, the following section will focus on the Vietnamese, Laotians, and Cambodians.

The main food staple in these countries is rice, which is eaten at most meals. The clothing differs, making it easy to distinguish a Vietnamese woman from a Cambodian woman; Vietnamese women wear long, flowing gowns over long pants, while Cambodian women wear long skirts wrapped around the waist. Laotian women wear long skirts with a distinctive border of intricate patterns. Vietnam is strongly influenced by China and France, and the majority of Vietnamese are either Buddhist or Catholic. Cambodia and Laos are influenced by India, and the majority of the people are Buddhists.

Indochinese languages are quite different. Vietnamese is tonal, and its writing system is alphabetical. Each lexeme is represented by a monosyllable. The Cambodian and Laotian languages are polysyllabic, and their writing systems are based on Sanskrit. All these languages have in common a rich lexicon of kinship terms, as all the cultures stress the central importance of the extended family and have elaborate kinship systems. Honorific terms are used to address the old, teachers, and authority figures.

Historical Perspective of Indochinese Immigration

Before 1975, there were very few Indochinese in the United States. The few that were in the country were generally university students. Since 1975, however, more than 1 million Indochinese have fled their countries because of Communist takeovers of their governments. The great exodus has continued to this day, and many of these refugees have come to the United States.

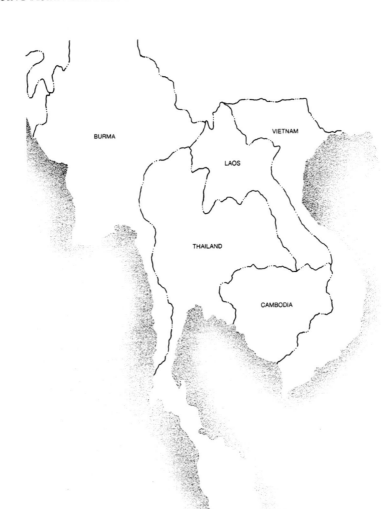

Figure 3-1 Indochina

Flight from Indochina

The first wave of Indochinese immigrants (refugees) came to the United States in 1975. They were Vietnamese who had either worked for or been affiliated with the U.S. government; they had been evacuated and airlifted out of Vietnam after Saigon fell to the Communists. They left for fear of persecution, many with only a moment's notice. Many left their families behind. It was a time of unrest, separation, anxiety, and fear. Many were taken to camps until their sponsors could arrange for their journey to the United States. These first refugees were educated and had some exposure to Western ideology and culture.

The second wave of refugees arrived between 1979 and 1982. This group included not only Vietnamese, but also Cambodians, Laotians, and Hmongs (many of whom are ethnic Chinese) who had escaped Indochina by land or by sea after the fall of South Vietnam. Many left their native countries on foot for the neighboring country of Thailand, and large refugee camps were set up along the border. Hundreds of thousands of refugees remained in the camps for months and years waiting for someone (family or friends) to sponsor them for immigration to other countries, such as the United States, Australia, and France. Hundreds of people escaped by cramming themselves onto small boats, thus earning the name "boat people." Approximately 50% of them perished at sea. Many starved to death. Some attempted to land in neighboring countries, but were refused entry. Others camped on deserted islands waiting to be rescued. Some Asian countries (e.g., Taiwan and Hong Kong) offered to take in some of the boat people, but the majority of them came to the United States.

On April 17, 1975, the Khmer Rouge moved into the capital of Cambodia. Within weeks, they were able to evacuate the cities and move the people into the countryside. Some Cambodians were put to hard labor and given very little food and shelter. Many were driven into the forest, some to die of starvation. Those who survived have recounted horrifying stories. They ate whatever they could find—worms, leaves, tree bark, spiders—until there was nothing left to eat. Corpses piled up along the roadside. Between 1975 and 1979, only the strongest managed to escape. After the Vietcong came into Cambodia in 1979, however, many were able to escape; they went to Thailand and, eventually, to other countries.

The second wave of refugees was quite different from the first. After 1975, there was no schooling in Vietnam and Cambodia, and only limited schooling in Laos. Thus, the second group of refugees tended to be less educated and to possess fewer job skills (Thuy, 1983). According to Buell (1985), these refugees were (1) less likely to be educated, (2) less likely to know English or other languages, (3) mainly rural, (4) likely to have been in camp for long periods of time (e.g., 3–5 years), and (5) likely to have had little or no contact with Western culture.

The third wave of refugees came after the Vietnamese government instituted the Orderly Departure Program (ODP) in 1982. The main purpose of this program is to allow the elderly, Amerasians, and unaccompanied minors to emigrate to the United States. These refugees are preliterate or illiterate. For more information about these people and their immigration into the United States, a list of suggested readings is provided in Appendix A.

Resettlement

The United Nations Commission for Refugees met in Geneva in 1978 to discuss the resettlement of the Indochinese refugees. Some countries offered places for permanent resettlement. The United States accepted the most refugees, followed by China, France, Canada, and Australia. Some countries offered financial assistance. Acting as sponsors themselves or finding a sponsor for each refugee, the voluntary resettlement agencies (Volags) help the refugees adjust to their new country.

The U.S. government has established numerous programs to assist refugees in their resettlement. For example, there are programs for English language training, vocational training, food stamps, and mental health centers. Many took advantage of the training programs and have become productive members of American society. For these refugees, life is stable and prosperous. They expect their children to finish school and to find gainful employment.

Other refugees have not adjusted so well. Some have had difficulty finding employment; some are underemployed, earning minimal wages, and cannot support their families. These refugees feel a sense of loss, isolation, and desperation. Many women must stay home to care for their children and lack the opportunity to receive language training. As a result, many feel segregated from the majority society. These circumstances may promote an unhappy and unstable home life for refugee families. Some of the youngsters feel alienated, powerless, and rejected. Some formed gangs when they were in the refugee camps and are now causing problems in the United States. Some have joined gangs and become juvenile delinquents since their arrival. These youngsters require guidance and counseling in order to feel accepted as a part of American society.

Anxiety and stress levels are high among refugees (Smither & Rodriguez-Giegling, 1979). In general, all face some degree of conflict with the new culture. Some learn to adapt and adjust to the new environment, becoming bicultural. They retain certain parts of the old culture and modify other parts in order to maintain their mental equilibrium. For those who cling to the old culture and fail to make adjustments, however, life in the new country can be difficult and unpleasant.

According to a recent study conducted by Nguyen and Henkin (1983), Vietnamese and Laotian refugees have perceived changes in their own cultural patterns since their resettlement. Vietnamese subjects noted a significant degree of change in the politeness and obedience of their children, the subordinate role of women, the (pre)dominant role of men, respect for older people, and the preservation of culture and customs. The Laotian group reported changes in the preservation of culture and customs, respect for older persons, the predominant role of men, conformity to the social order, the filial piety ethic, and the subordinate role of women. The Vietnamese subjects considered these changes to be negative, while the Laotian group viewed the changes as relatively positive. Because it is "often difficult to get a Lao to give a frank opinion" (Bar, 1960, p. 98) and because Laotians have a tendency toward "tacit acquiescence" (Nguyen & Henkin, 1983, p. 169), the findings on the Laotian subjects may not be totally reliable. Nguyen and Henkin suggested that "programs that serve to facilitate social adaptation while allowing sufficient latitude to accommodate significant cultural differences are likely to have a higher level of success" (p. 169).

Religion

The primary religion in Vietnam, Laos, and Cambodia is Buddhism. The Vietnamese culture is also heavily influenced by the Confucian tradition. In addition, people in various parts of Indochina, specifically the highland Laotian people, practice animism. Believing that everything has a spirit, even a tree, they build temples and roadside shrines where they worship these spirits. They also believe that there are a number of wandering spirits and they pay their respects to these spirits in special ceremonies. Furthermore, the Indochinese show respect for their ancestors by holding special ceremonies in their memory.

The Vietnamese

Most Vietnamese are Buddhists, the remainder being Confucianists, Catholics, and Taoists. The Taoist metaphysical concept of harmony, the Confucian ethical and social principles, and the Buddhist theory of reincarnation and act retribution have been blended together into a form of philosophy and religion known as the "Three Teachings." They constitute the foundation of all traditions, customs, and manners of the Vietnamese people.

Historical Background

The ethnic Vietnamese are believed to be descendants of Mongols who moved south and spread over the Red River delta. The Chinese ruled Vietnam for 1,000 years before the first Vietnamese dynasty was established in 938 A.D. Between 938 A.D. and 1776 A.D., Vietnam was a colony of China. In 1776, the country was divided in half, with the Nguyen dynasty ruling in the South and the Trinh dynasty ruling in the North. In 1867, the southern portion of Vietnam was taken by the French, who called it Cochinchina. In 1882, the French seized Hanoi; between 1887 and 1893, they created a union that included Tonkin, Annam, Cochinchina, Cambodia, and Laos, calling it French Indochina. The French ruled French Indochina until 1945, when the Japanese overthrew the French authorities and granted independence to Vietnam. After the Japanese surrendered at the end of World War II, however, the French regained control. When Vietnamese attempts to negotiate with the French for independence failed, the French-Indochinese war began. It ended in 1954 when the Vietnamese defeated the French at the battle of Dien Bien Phu. Under the 1954 Geneva Accord, Vietnam was divided along the 17th parallel, into North and South Vietnam.

In the early 1960s, the Vietcong started to penetrate South Vietnam. After 1964, the war intensified, and the United States became heavily involved. Finally, a peace agreement was signed in Paris in 1973. After the U.S. forces were withdrawn, the Vietcong continued its infiltration of troops into South Vietnam, and Saigon fell into Communist hands on April 30, 1975. This resulted in a massive evacuation and uprooting of more than 100,000 Vietnamese.

The Vietnamese Language

As mentioned earlier, Vietnamese is a tonal language that is basically monosyllabic. In the early part of the 20th century, after the French occupation in the late 19th century, the Vietnamese adopted a modified Romanized alphabet system to replace the old writing system that had been derived from Chinese characters (Exhibit 3-1). Diacritical marks are used to signify the tone of each word. This system remains in use today.

The tones with the pitch changes within a word reflect different lexical meanings (Table 3-1). Vietnamese includes many words derived from other languages, such as English, French, Malay, and Chinese. For example, the word *mit-tinh* has its origin in the English word *meeting;* its meaning has evolved and become demonstration. The word *xa-rông* is borrowed from the Malay word *sarong,* which means a type of wrap-around clothing; the word *xà-bông* is borrowed from the French word *savon,* which means soap; and the word *bacsi* is taken from the Chinese word 博士, which means doctor.

English vs. Vietnamese Phonetic Systems

A comparative analysis of the English and Vietnamese phonetic systems reveals the following differences (Vietnamese consonants and vowels are found in Tables 3-2 and 3-3):

1. Consonant blends occur in all word positions (i.e., initial, medial, and final) in English, whereas there are no consonant blends in Vietnamese.
2. Syllabic stress is used for contrastive purposes in English, but is not phonemic in Vietnamese. Lexemes in Vietnamese are typically monosyllabic.

Exhibit 3-1 Vietnamese Alphabet

Letter	Phonetic Value (IPA symbols)	Key Word and Meaning
VOWELS		
i	i	đị: go
y		biêt-ly: separation
e	ɛ	nghe: hear
ê	e	lê : pear
a	a	ba: three
ă	ɐ	bắp: corn
â	ʌ	lân: unicorn
u	u	đu: swing
u'	ɯ	thu': letter
o	ɔ	to: big
ô	o	tôm: shrimp
o'	ɤ	mo': dream
CONSONANTS		
b	b	bi: marble
p	p	bắọ: corn
c, k	k	cá: fish ,kim: needle
ch	c	cha: father
d	z (Northern dialect)	de: goat
	j (Central & Southern)	
đ	d	điêc: deaf
g ,gh	g	{ gân: near
		{ ghét: hate
h	h	ho: cough
kh	x	khinh: despise
l	l	la: shout
m	m	me: mother
n	n	ninh: flatter
nh	ɲ	nh'à: house
ng,ngh	ŋ	ngà: ivory
		nghe: hear
gi	z (Northern)	già: old
	j (Southern & Central)	
ph	f	phai: fade
q	kw	quên: forget
r	{ z Northern	ruôi: flies
	{ ʒ Central & Southern	
	{ r in some dialects (Northern, Central and Southern)	
s	{ ʃ Central & Southern	sao: star
	{ s (Northern & some Southern dialects)	
t	t	tên: name
th	t'	thu: autumn
tr	{ t Central & Southern	trâu: water buffalo
	{ c (Northern)	
v	{ v Central & Northern	voi: elephant
	{ j Southern	
x	s	xa: far

Source: Used with permission of Huynh Dinh Te.

Table 3-1 Significance of Tones in Vietnamese Vowels

Tone	Vietnamese Word	Lexical Meaning
1. Level	ma	Ghost
2. Breathing rising	má	Cheek, mommy
3. Breathing falling	mà	But
4. Falling rising	mã	Tomb
5. Creaky rising (low rising)	mã	Horse
6. Low falling (low constricted)	ma̱	Rice seedling
1. Level	la	Short
2. Breathing rising	lá	Leaf
3. Breathing falling	là	To be
4. Falling rising	lã	Exhausted
5. Creaky rising	lã	Plain water
6. Low falling	la̱	Stranger
1. Level	ba	Three
2. Breathing rising	bá	Cypress tree
3. Breathing falling	bà	Grandmother
4. Falling rising	bã	Bait
5. Creaky rising	bã	Residue
6. Low falling	ba̱	Bad, wrong

3. English uses many final consonants; however, Vietnamese uses only a limited number of final consonants, including /p/, /t/, /k/, /m/, /n/, and /ŋ/.

Possible Phonetic Interferences for Vietnamese Speakers

Vietnamese speakers who are learning English may mispronounce certain English phonemes by substituting a similar Vietnamese phoneme. Exhibit 3-2 (Te, 1984) is the contrastive analysis of the Vietnamese and the English vowel and consonant systems. Possible phonetic interferences of the Vietnamese language for Vietnamese speakers who are learning English are shown in Table 3-4.

The Laotians

Laos is situated south of China, north of Cambodia, east of Thailand and Burma, and west of Vietnam. It is 850 kilometers long and 50 to 350 kilometers wide. Two-thirds of Laos is jungle. It is a tropical country with an average annual rainfall of 70 inches. There is a dry season from November to April and a wet season from May to October. The Mekong River provides fish and serves as the major transportation route.

Historical Background

According to oral Laotian history which dates back to 3000 B.C. (there was no written history before the 14th century), the Laotian people originally lived in the Yunnan area of China, but they settled in Laos in the 6th century A.D. The first Kingdom of Laos was established in the mid-14th century and by the 17th century had expanded to include some territory that is now part of Thailand, Vietnam, and Cambodia. Before 1707, the country was split into three major kingdoms. The King of Thailand took over Laos in 1779. As part of French Indochina, Laos was under the French rule between 1893 and 1954. Japan occupied Laos for a short period during World War II, but France regained control in

Table 3-2 Vietnamese Consonants

Sounds (IPA Symbols)	Spelling	Key Words		Distribution Initial	Final
p	p		dẹp(pretty)		x
b	b	ba(three)		x	
t	t	tai(ear)	hát(sing)	x	x(Northern)
t'	th	thư'(letter)		x	
d	d	den(black)		x	
ţ	tr	tre(bamboo)		x	
c	ch	cha(father)	sách(book)	x	x(Southern and Central)
k	c, k	ca(sing) ký(sign)	bác(uncle)	x	x
k͡p	c		học (study)		x
g	g, gh	gan(liver) ghét(hate)		x	
m	m	ma(ghost)	im(silent)	x	x
n	n	nó(he/she)	lan(orchid)	x	x(Northern)
ɲ	nh	nhà(house)	lính(soldier)	x	x(Southern and Central)
ŋ	ng, ngh	ngà(ivory) nghe(hear)	làng (village)	x	x
ŋ͡m	ng		lông(hair)		x
f	ph	phí(waste)		x	
v	v	v'ê(go back)		x (not in Southern)	
s	x	xa(far)		x	
z	d, gi, r	rong(seaweed) da(skin) già(old)		x (in Northern only)	
ʃ	s	sai(wrong)		x (not in Northern)	
3	r	r'ông(dragon)		x (not in Northern)	
j	d, gi	da(skin) già(old)		x (not in Northern)	
x	kh	khen(praise)		x	
h	h	hè(summer)		x	
l	l	lê(pear)		x	
r	r	ru'ôi(fly)		x (in some dialects only)	
w	u, o	oà(burst out crying) hoa(flower) quý(precious)		x	medialx
y	i	hai(two)		x	x

1946. In 1949, France granted independence to Laos. In 1973, the royal Laotian government and the Communist Pathet Lao reached an accord. Later, in 1975, the Communist government established the Democratic Republic of Laos.

Soon after the fall of South Vietnam and the Vietcong invasion, many Laotians were sent to reeducation camps established by the Pathet Lao and the Vietcong to promote Communist doctrines. Many Laotians feared for their lives and attempted to escape. Some tried to escape by boat or by swimming across the river to the three or four Laotian refugee camps across the border in neighboring Thailand. At the present time, there are more than 100,000 Laotians in these refugee camps, where there is a great shortage of food and medical supplies. A family of four may share a space of no more than 144 square feet. Food and

Table 3-3 Vietnamese Vowels

Sounds (IPA Symbols)	Spelling	Key Words	Initial	Medial	Final
i	i	im(silent) tim(heart) di(go)	x	x	x
e	ê	êm(soft,smooth) tên(name) lê(pear)	x	x	x
ɛ	e	em(younger sibling) tem(stamp) nghe(hear)	x	x	x
a	a	am(small temple) tám(eight) ma(ghost)	x	x	x
u	u	út(youngest child) cút(quail) thu(autumn)	x	x	x
ɯ	u'	u'a(like) xu'a(old) thu'(letter)	x	x	x
o	ô	ôm(hug) tôm(shrimp) xô(push)	x	x	x
ɤ	ơ	ơn (favor) lời(word) tơ(silk)	x	x	x
ɔ	o	ói(throw up) xóm(hamlet) to(big)	x	x	x
ɐ	ă	ăn(eat) xăng(gasoline)	x	x	
ʌ	â	âḿ(warm) cãm(forbid)	x	x	

Source: Used with permission of Huynh Dinh Te.

water are rationed, and people wait in long lines for supplies. The average length of stay is 3 years. Many stay for 4, 5, or 6 years until they can be relocated. Some of the camp people have organized schools for the young children.

Traditionally, Laotian names are names of objects or words with special meaning. Family names were not considered important until 1943 when the French instituted mandatory adoption of family names.

The population of Laos in 1975 was 3.5 million. The great exodus that followed the Communist takeover drastically reduced the population of Laos; it is now approximately 2 million. Of these, 50% are Laotians; 16%, Thais; and 5%, Hmong. The remainder of the population includes Yius, Mienhs, and Kais.

Only 35% of Laotians were literate. Those who did go to school learned French and English. Because many of the Laotian refugees lack basic literacy skills, never having learned to read or write in their native language, they find it extremely difficult to learn English. Without language skills in English, they find it difficult to obtain training and employment in the United States.

Major cultural differences also contribute to the adjustment problems of Laotians who have resettled in the United States. As do all Asians, the Laotians revere the old. They have large families, and extended families are not uncommon. The nursing home is a foreign concept to them, and they are shocked that

Exhibit 3-2 Contrastive Analysis of English and Vietnamese Vowel and Consonant Systems

(IPA symbols)

English Vowels / Vowel Nuclei	seat / i	sit / I	bed / e	bad / æ	car / ɑ	fall / ɔ	fool / u	full / ʊ	love / ə	day / ei	five / ai	house / aʊ	boy / ɔt	know / oʊ	here / Iə	hair / ɛɚ	poor / ʊə	fire / aia	hour / aʊa
English	x	x	x	x	x	x	x	x	x	x	x	x	x	x	x	x	x	x	x
Vietnamese	x		x̣		x̣	x	x		x̣	x̣	x	x	(x)	x̣	x̣	(x)	x		

English Consonants	pin / p	boy / b	ten / t	dog / d	cat / k	get / g	chair / +ʃ	just / dʒ	man / m	not / n	sing / ŋ	fan / f	van / v	thank / θ	this / ð	sow / s	his / z	show / ʃ	pleasure / ʒ	red / r	hot / h	lane / ℓ
Initial — English	x	x	x	x	x	x	x	x	x	x		x	x	x	x	x	x	x		x	x	x
Initial — Vietnamese		x	x̣	x	x̣	x̣			x	x	x	x	(x)			x	(x)	(x)	(x)	(x̣)	x	x
Medial — English	x	x	x	x	x	x	x	x	x	x	x	x	x	x	x	x	x	x	x	x	x	x
Medial — Vietnamese																						
Final — English	x	x	x	x	x	x	x	x	x	x	x	x	x	x	x	x	x	x	x	x		x
Final — Vietnamese	x̣		x̣		x̣				x̣	x̣	x̣											

Note: (x): not occurring in all dialects of Vietnamese
x̣ : having different articulation from English sounds
Source: Used with permission of Huynh Dinh Te.

Table 3-4 Possible Phonetic Interferences of Vietnamese in Learning English

Interference	Sound	Example
Distortion	/c+ʃh/	church
	/dʒz/	juice
Substitution	k/kl	cass/class
	t/t	tie/tie
	p/p'	pie/pie
	s/ʃ	sue/shoe
	s/tʃ	sue/chew
Omission of final consonant	/p/	to/top
	/d/	bu/bud
	/g/	do/dog
	/tʃ/	cat/catch
	/dʒ/	ju/judge
	/f/	kni/knife
	/v/	fi/five
	/θ/	ma/math
	/ð/	brea/breathe
	/s/	offi/office
	/z/	wa/was
	/ʃ/	ma/mash
	/ʒ/	rou/rouge
	/r/	ca/car
	/l/	ca/call

old people are sent away to such facilities. Parents have a hard time coping with the changes that rapidly appear in their children; many do not cope well and suffer deep depression.

Laotian Culture

The Laotian refugees bring with them their many customs and beliefs. Most Laotians are Buddhist, and most Laotian men are required to spend 2 or 3 weeks as a monk before they marry. Many believe in the practice of folk medicine and the ritual of Baci. Believing that every human being has 32 souls, many Laotians ask a sorcerer to perform this ritual to call back the souls of a person who is sick in order to bring about that person's recovery. Because the king of souls is believed to reside in a person's head, the head is considered a sacred area and should not be touched. The ceremony of Baci is also conducted for farewell parties and births, and the sorcerer prays to every god and spells the magic words on silk strings that are tied to the individual.

Teachers working with Laotian children need to become familiar with the Laotian way of life in order to understand the children's behavior. For example, Laotian students generally do not say, "I don't know," believing that it is a sign of disrespect for the teacher. Similarly, they rarely say, "no," because they think that saying no will hurt the teacher's feelings. They generally do not look the teacher in the eye, because staring is regarded as a sign of challenge, disrespect, and aggression. Pointing at people is considered very impolite, and touching the opposite sex is unacceptable. Parents regard the school as a safe place and feel that the teachers have absolute knowledge.

As these people go through the process of acculturation, they become more accustomed to the American way of schooling. The degree of acculturation depends on the amount of exposure these people have to the Western behavioral patterns.

The Laotian Language

Most Laotian words are monosyllabic, although there are some compound and polysyllabic words borrowed from Sanskrit and Pali, two languages from India. These polysyllabic words relate to Buddhism, science, and philosophy. The Laotian alphabet is also adapted from Sanskrit and Pali. It is a system in which there are more symbols than sounds. Unlike English, Laotian has almost no exceptions to the sound-symbol correspondences. Like Chinese and Vietnamese, Laotian is tonal. The "Vietiane" dialect is considered the standard dialect. It has six tones, namely (1) high, (2) rising, (3) rising-falling, (4) falling-rising, (5) falling, and (6) short. Syllable types include consonant-vowel-consonant (CVC), consonant-vowel-vowel-consonant (CVVC), and consonant-vowel-vowel (CVV).

The Laotian lexicon is quite complex in that different sets of lexical items are used in conversations with people of different social status. For example, there are seven different words that a Laotian may use to refer to himself, depending on whether he is talking to (1) a Buddha or a monk, (2) a monarch, (3) a mandarin, (4) a high civil servant or a military officer, (5) an ordinary person on the street, (6) a close friend, or (7) a person to whom hostility is expressed. All seven of the terms translate into English as I, since there is only one word *I* in English. In order to address people appropriately and use appropriate language, however, Laotian speakers must determine the listener's relative social rank. When this is not clear, they are uneasy about responding.

Although the language uses five different tones to denote syllables and the individual words have their tonemes, there is no stress in the Laotian. As a result, the language sounds monotonous, and speakers of Laotian have difficulty in placing primary and secondary stress on polysyllabic English words they have learned. Furthermore, as most Laotian words end in a vowel, English final consonants are difficult for Laotians to produce (Table 3-5).

The basic order of words in a Laotian sentence is similar to that of an English sentence: subject + verb + object. Subjects are often omitted in Laotian, however. There are other morphological and syntactical differences between English and Laotian:

- Adjectives follow nouns in Laotian, for example, dress that have color good.
- Personal pronouns do not change in Laotian. There is only one word for the words *I*, *me*, *my*, and *mine*. Moreover, there is no gender differentiation in third person singular pronouns.
- In Laotian, the meaning of plurality and possession is expressed with different combinations of words, rather than with markers.
- There are no tense markers in Laotian. The meaning of past, present, or future is expressed through the words of time in the sentence. For example, I go school yesterday.

Table 3-5 Possible Phonetic Interferences of Laotian in Learning English

Interferences	Sound	Example
Omission of final consonant	/b/	bi/bib
	/d/	di/did
	/g/	do/dog
	/f/	kni/knife
	/v/	wa/wave
	/l/	ba/ball
	/s/	ni/nice
Confusion of vowels	i/I	eat/it
	o/ɔ	boat/bought
	e/ɛ	sat/set
	e/æ	satan/satin
	u/v	food/foot
Difficulty in producing consonant blends	/sp-/	pell/spell
	/sm-/	mall/small
	/pr-/	pay/pray
	/bl-/	bend/blend
	/pt/	ap/apt
	/-nd/	an/and
	/-the/	cloth/clothes
Substitution of consonants	p/b	bip/bib
	t/d	bet/bed
	p/f	leap/leaf
	p/v	lop/love
	t/s	bat/bass
	n/l	pin/pill
	w/v (F)	warve/wave

- A Laotian verb does not change its form when there is a change in subject. For example, I go, you go, he go.
- Laotian has no verb *to be* for sentences with predicate adjectives, for example, food good, dress beautiful.
- There are no articles in Laotian.
- The word *bo* used in the beginning of a Laotian sentence indicates negation.
- The same word *bo*, when placed at the end of a sentence, becomes a question marker. There is no change in word order when the sentence is an interrogative. For example, do you want to go?/pai bo?; you don't want to go/bo pai; and/don't you want to go?/bo pai bo?

The Hmong

Originally from China, the Hmong moved to the mountainous area of Indochina centuries ago. They are scattered throughout China, Thailand, Laos, Burma, and Vietnam. They have a rich oral history of legends and folktales that have been passed down from one generation to the next. People in Asia refer to them as Meo, Miao, or Miau. Other spellings include Mung, Muong, H'mong, Hmoob, and Hmuong. Only recently has a written language been developed, however.

Between 1960 and 1975, thousands of Hmong were recruited by the Central Intelligence Agency (CIA) to conduct clandestine maneuvers in the region against the Vietcong and the Communist Pathet Lao (Walker, 1985). After the fall of South Vietnam in 1975, approximately 100,000 fled to escape retaliation for these activities. Most of them had never been outside their mountain homeland before their evacuation. The majority of them were illiterate. Prior to their uprooting, they had not been exposed to the conveniences (and stresses) of the "modern world." Thus, the Hmong who resettled in the United States faced tremendous problems.

There are approximately 60,000 Hmong now living in the United States. In some cases, they have become unwelcomed aliens of the American cities in which they settled. Most of them have congregated in the so-called Indochinese communities, the de facto Indochinese ghettos. Anthropologists have observed that displaced national groups cling most stubbornly to three principal cultural attributes: language, typical or accustomed foods, and religion. The elderly Hmong in the United States practice folk medicine and continue to perform indigenous religious rituals. They wear native costumes and eat ethnic foods. An agrarian people, the Hmong prefer to grow their own vegetables, and they find it extremely difficult to adjust to an urban life style that makes it impossible for them to continue their customary way of life. The immense social and psychological upheaval that the older Hmong have experienced has left them physically and financially dependent on their children, physically and psychologically isolated, without self-esteem, and with few skills necessary for life in American mainstream society (*Refugee Update*, 1985).

In a study of Hmong communities, Meredith and Cramer (1982) found that 92% of those interviewed reported stress-related illnesses. Many of them have tried to learn English and to obtain vocational training without success. Studies indicate that at least 75% of the refugees are not employed, and most are receiving government assistance. They have difficulty learning to use modern home appliances, such as the refrigerator, washer and dryer, stove, and toilet; many have continued their old customs, drying fish in their living rooms, hanging clothes on tree branches, and making fires for cooking in the living room. They are homesick, experiencing tremendous "culture shock" and not adjusting very well. Of the Hmong interviewed by Smalley (1985), 65% said that life in the United States was not better than life in Laos was, and 86% said that they would return to Laos if they could. Only 10% said that they would stay in the United States if they had an opportunity to return to Laos (Dowling, Hendricks, Mason, & Olney, 1984).

Efforts have been made by some institutions, including Yale University, to collect and publish papers and essays about the Hmong culture. The Hmong themselves have begun to publish *Haiv Hmong*, a Hmong language journal, in order to establish links among the Hmong scattered throughout the United States and to preserve the Hmong heritage. The first issue of the journal called in English *The Hmong World* was published in 1986. It contained articles on Shamanism, changes in tradition, White Hmong kinship terminology, and sung poetry. It was published by Yale Southeast Asian Studies, Box 13A, Yale Station, New Haven, CT 06520.

Sound System of Hmong

The Hmong language is a Sino-Tibetan language. There are two variations: White and Blue/Green. It has the following phonemic characteristics:

1. Several consonant sounds such as /p/, /t/, /r/, /ty/, /qh/, /ts/, and /t/, have both aspirated and unaspirated forms.
2. /r/ is a stop rather than a liquid. Tongue placement is approximately midpalate. Aspirated /r/ may sound like English /t/, while unaspirated /r/ may sound like English /d/.
3. The only final consonant is /ŋ/.
4. Consonant clusters, which occur only in initial positions, include nasals + stops (e.g., /np/, /nt/, and /nts/) and nasals + stops + /e/ (e.g., /npl/).
5. w is /+/ in White Hmong and /ü/ in Blue/Green Hmong. No vowels are reduced to /ę/ schwa.
6. /d/ exists in White Hmong, but not Blue/Green Hmong.

These phonemic characteristics may create certain difficulties for Hmongs who are trying to learn English (Table 3-6). There are 32 consonants in White Hmong and 28 in Blue/Green Hmong.

White Hmong	Aspirated	ph [p']	th [t']	rh [t']	ch [ty']
	Unaspirated	p [p]	t [t]	r [t]	c [ty]
	Aspirated	kh [k']	gh [k']	txh [ts']	tsh [ch']
	Unaspirated	k [k]	g [k]	tx [ts]	ts [ch]
		f [f]	x [s]	z [zh]	y [y]
		v [v]	xy [sy]	s [sh]	h [h]
		m [m]	n [n]	ny [ñ]	
		hm [hm]	hn [hn]	hny [hñ]	
		ℓ [ℓ]			
		hℓ [hℓ]			

Note: ? = Roman Popular Alphabet

[] = Pronunciation.

Table 3-6 Possible Phonetic Interferences of Hmong in Learning English

Interferences	Sound	Example
Difficulty with consonant clusters, except for /pl/ and /bl/		
Omission of final consonants, except for /y/		
Substitution	+ʃ/ʃ	chair/share
	d/dʒ	drive/juice
	ℓ/r	light/right
	z/ð	zis/this
	s/θ	sum/thumb
Difficulty with vowels	/I/	
	/i/	
	/o/	
	/ʊ/	
	/ə/	

Blue/Green Hmong does not have the [hm]-[m], [hn]-[n], [hñ]-[ñ] distinctions. Furthermore, the Blue/Green Hmong use [tℓ] [t'ℓ] [dℓ] but not [dh] [d] [nd].

Vowel System

There are six basic vowels in Hmong:

i, i, u, ey, ɔ, a

White Hmong has two nasal vowels and five diphthongs:

ong, eng, and ia, ua, ai, au, ət

Blue/Green Hmong has the following:

ü, əü, ẽ, õ, ã

Tones

There are seven tones in Hmong.

Tone Description	Number	Example
high	1	pob [pɔ¹] 'lump'
high falling	2	poj [pɔ²] 'female'
mid-rising	3	pov [pɔ³] 'throw'
mid	4	po [pɔ⁴] 'pancreas'
low	5	pos [pɔ⁵] 'thorn'
low breathing	6	pog [pɔ⁶] 'paternal grandfather'
short low abrupt end	7	pom [pɔ⁷] 'see'

The Cambodians

Almost all Cambodians speak Khmer, a language of the Austro-Asiatic language family. Many other languages are also spoken in Cambodia, namely, Chinese, Vietnamese, Thai, Cahm, Laotian, and Indian. French, however, is the language of the educated class and is used to communicate with the outside world. Thus, the rural population of Cambodia is predominantly monolingual, while urban Cambodians are generally bilingual or trilingual. The speech of Phnom Penh, the capital, varies slightly from the speech of the other provinces.

India has had an important influence on the Khmer language and culture. The Khmer alphabet was derived from the alphabets of Sanskrit, the language of Hinduism, and Pali, the religious language of Buddhism. The written system of Khmer has two forms: Aksar Mul (full letter) and Aksar Crieng (leaning letter). The full letter form is used for sacred texts, headlines, and inscriptions on monuments and public buildings, and the leaning letter form is used for everyday correspondence and documents.

In order to address different groups of people appropriately, the people in Cambodia use four different forms of Khmer: the language of the ordinary people, the formal language, the language of the clergy, and the royal language (Table 3-7). Furthermore, Khmer speakers use numerous terms of address:

1. I
   - /Khñom/ The usual and neutral form, this term is used to address an elderly person or someone of the same rank. It is a safe and polite word for foreigners to use, except to monks and royalty.
   - / ɔñ/ This term is used to address children or someone who is intimate with the speaker. It is impolite to use this word to address an elderly person.
   - /Khñom Bat/ This term is used by men when speaking to superiors, parents, and elderly people.
   - /Nl:əng Khñom/ This term is used by women when speaking to superiors, parents, and elderly people.
   - /Khñom Preh Kɔrona/ This term is used by laymen when they address a monk.
   - /Nì:anɔ/ Khñom Preh Kɔrona/ This term is used by laywomen when they address a monk.
   - /Tùl Preh Bɔngkum CÌ:əkhñom/ This term is used by a commoner to address the king.
2. you
   - /Nèək/ This term is used among friends of both sexes. It is both familiar and polite; it is also used by husband and wife.
   - /Nèək ʔaeng/ This term is used to show respect to the addressee.
   - /ʔaeng/ This term is used when friends of the same age are talking together.

Table 3-7 Examples of Different Forms of Khmer

Meaning	Ordinary People	Formal Relationships	Clergy	Royalty
Eat	/Si:/	/Pisa:/	/Chan/	/Saoy/
Go	/Təu/	/Pan cə̀: ñ/	/Nimun/	/Yi: ng/
Drink	/phək/	/Pisa:/	/Chan/	/Saoy/
Sleep	/De:k/	/Samran:n/	/sə̀ng/	/Phtùm/
Die	/Slap/	/Mə̀:rə̀:nak/	/Sokùt/	/Sokùt/
To be born	/Kaət/	/Kaət/	/Kaət/	/Pr :sot/
Give	/Aoy/	/Cu:ən/	/Prə̀:kè:n/	/Thvay/
Speak	/Niyì:əy/	/Mi:ən Prə̀:sah/	/Mi:ən Puth:dəyka/	/Mi:ən Prèh Pən tùl/

3. we
   - /Yə̀:ng/ This is the general neutral term.
   - /ʔaeng. ʔ ʊ ñ/ This term (i.e., you and I) is used in conversation with a close friend.
   - /Yə̀:ng Khñom/ This term is more polite than /Yə̀:ng/. It is also used when the speaker is one of the group referred to (i.e., I and the other).
4. he, she, they
   - /Kɛ̆ə̀t/ This term is used to refer to people for whom the speaker feels respect.
   - /Kè:/ This term is used for people in general (i.e., they say . . .).
   - /Vì:ə̀/ This term is used to refer to children, animals, and things.
5. other terms of address
   - /Lòk/ This term (i.e., Mr., Sir) is used between equals (men) who speak formally to each other.
   - /Lò:ksrə̀y/ This term (i.e., Ms., Mrs., Madame) is used between women who speak formally to each other. It is also used in conversation with a married woman of high rank.
   - /Nɛ̆ə̀ksrə̀y/ This term (i.e., Ms., Mrs., Madame) is used to refer to a married woman of the middle class.
   - /Nì:ə̀ng/ This term (i.e., Miss, young) is used for formally addressing girls and young women up to 20 years old of any rank. It may also be used to address both boys and girls up to 13 years old politely, yet affectionately.
   - /B>:ng, O:n/ This term (i.e., brother, sister) is used in the affectionate speech of husband to wife and vice versa.

Unlike Vietnamese and Laotian, Khmer is not a tonal language. Like English, it has overall sentential intonation patterns. Simple, affirmative, negative, and interrogative statements are characterized by a steep fall in intonation on the final syllable.

Khmer words are usually monosyllabic or dissyllabic, whereby stress always falls on the second syllable. The syllable types include the following combinations of consonants (C) and vowels (V): CVC, CCVC, CCCVC, CVVC, CCVVC, CCCVVC, CVV, CCVV (e.g., Can/dish, Krong/city, Phtùk/load, and Khmeng/child).

The few polysyllabic words in Khmer are either compound words or words derived from another language. Compound words may be regular compound words

| Sokh Sɔbbay | fine |
| fine happy | |

or technical compound words, such as those formed with Tuɾ (far)

Tuɾrle:k	telegram
far number	
Tuɾsaph	
far sound	telephone
Tuɾtɔ:sn	
far vision	television
Tuɾk ɔ:m	
far communication	telecommunication

Table 3-8 Khmer Consonant Chart

	Nonaspirated	Aspirated	Nonaspirated	Aspirated	Nasal
Velar	/K/	/KH/	/K̇/	/KḢ/	/NĠ/
Palatal	/C/	/CH/	/Ċ/	/CḢ/	/NḢ/
Retroflex (dental)	/D/	/TH/	/Ḋ/	/TḢ/	/Ṅ/
Dental	/T/	/TH/	/Ṫ/	/TḢ/	/Ṅ/
Labial	/B/	/PH/	/Ṗ/	/PḢ/	/Ṁ/
Continuants I	/Ẏ/	/Ṙ/	/L̇/	/V̇/	(All second register)
Continuants II	/S/	/H/	/L/	/ð/	(All first register)

Most technical lexical items in Khmer have been derived from French. Many common words also have French origins, however, such as bière (beer), cafe (coffee), aeroplane (airplane), posté (post office), timbre (stamp), and marful (mark). Similarly, many Khmer words have been derived from Sanskrit (Table 3-9).

The Khmer consonant chart is presented in Table 3-8. There are 85 different initial consonant clusters in Khmer. Most, but not all, are very different from those of the English language (e.g., Mtyul, and Sdap, but Knog). Khmer stops /p/, /t/, /k/, /ʔ/, and /c/ are both aspirated and nonaspirated. There are only two

Table 3-9 Khmer Words Derived from Sanskrit

	Khmer		Sanskrit	
Meaning	Writing	Pronunciation	Writing	Pronunciation
Son		/Botra/		/Putra/
Friend		/Mitt/		/Mitra/
Father		/Bʏyda/		/Pita/
Mother		/Mì:ðda/		/Matha/
Daughter		/Thi:da/		/Dhītā/
Love		/Snaeha/		/Snehā/
Sin		/Kamm/		/Kamma/
Festival		/Bony/		/Punya/
Heart		/Cett/		/Chitta/
Life		/Cì:vi:t/		/Jīvita/
Girl		/Komarʏy/		/Kumārī/
Temple		/Vihì:ɔ·r/		/Vihāra/
Renown		/Kʏtteyùɔ·s/		/Kittiyasa/
Behavior		/Keriya:/		/Kiriȳa/
Pity		/Karuna:/		/Karunā/
Time		/Samay/		/Samaya/
Go		/Yi:ɔtra/		virgule Yātrā/

Table 3-10 Possible Phonetic Interferences of Khmer in Learning English

Interference	Sound
Substitutions	k/g
	v/w
	f/b
	tʃ/ʃ
	z/ɗ,d/ɗ
	s/θ
	t/θ
Approximation	Khmer palatal
	trill r/
	English r
Omission of final	
consonants	r
	d
	g
	s
	b
	z
Vowel distortion	ɛ, i, ɪ, ʊ, æ
Implosive sound	/b/
	/d/

fricatives in Khmer. The Khmer vowels are divided into short and long vowels. These phonetic differences often cause Khmer speakers to make certain errors in speaking English (Table 3-10).

    Khmeng Pì:r   two children
    Khmeng Khlah   some children

Similarly, Khmer verbs remain unchanged in different linguistic contexts:

    Khñom Sdap Phlè:ng   I hear the music.
      I   hear music
    Kè: Sdap Phlè:ng   He hears the music.
    He hear music

    The verb *to be* in English has an equivalent in Khmer; however, it occurs in specific linguistic contexts. For example, the sentence *Sok is a doctor* is expressed as

    Sok Cì:ə; Krù: Pè:t
    Sok is   doctor

in Khmer. The sentence *My friend is fat* is expressed

    Mitt Khñom Thùm
    friend my   fat

and the sentence *I am at home* is expressed as

    Khñom Nə̀u Phtèh.
      I   at home

The following are some of the other syntactical characteristics of Khmer:

- Negative statements are formed by placing the following words immediately before the main verb: Min (not), Et (no), Pum (do not), and Kmì:ən (have not). The word *Tè* is a final negative marker:

Khñom Tə̀u Sala   I go to school.
  I   go school
Khñom Min Tə̀u Sala Tè   I do not go to school.
  I   not   go school

- Interrogative statements are formed by placing at the beginning of the statement the word *Taə̀*, which corresponds to the English auxiliary *do*, for example, Taə̀Neə̀k Tə̀u Sala Tè (Do you go to school?). The word *Tè* is used as a final interrogative marker as well.
- Table 3-11 shows the use of personal pronouns in Khmer.
- Khmer has progressive, past, and future tense markers:

Khñom Kampong Tə̀u   I am going.
  I   now   go
Khñom Ban Tə̀u Haə̀y   I have gone already.
  I   already go
Khñom Nwìng Tə̀u   I will go.
  I   future go

Table 3-11   Use of Personal Pronouns in Khmer

	English		Khmer	
Subject	I	I go to school.	Khñom	/Khñom Tə̀u Sala/ I go school
Object	Me	You tell me.	Khñom	/Neə̀k Prap Khñom/ You tell me
Possessive adjective	My + noun	I have my car.	Noun & Khñom	/Khñom Mì:ɤ n Lan Khñom I have car my
Possessive pronoun	Mine	This is mine.	R :b s Khñom (belong to)	/Neh Cì:ɤ Rɔ:bɔs Khñom/ this is mine
Reflexive	Myself	I cut myself.	Khlù: n Khñom (body)	/Khñom Cat Khlù:ɤ n Khñom/ I cut myself

---

Conclusion

Indochinese refugees have had to face devastating changes in their lives. Many have lost all that is familiar and now find themselves in the United States, confronted by a bewildering array of strange places, people, and things. In order to become comfortable and successful in their new lives, they must learn a new language—English. The speech-language-hearing clinician who knows the history of these refugees, the basic principles of their own linguistic systems, and the features of English most difficult for them to master can facilitate the learning process.

CHAPTER 4

Other Asians:
The Filipinos, Koreans, Japanese, Hawaiians, Guamanians, and Micronesians

The Filipinos

The Philippines is an archipelago of more than 7,200 islands situated south of China and southeast of Indochina. The country is slightly larger than the state of Arizona. Its weather is tropical, and there are many typhoons in the summer. Ninety-five percent of the population are of Malayan origin. Other racial and cultural influences include the Chinese, Spanish, aborigine, Amerasian, and Japanese.

Historical Background

Before 1521, the Philippines was a sovereign state that traded with China and many other Eastern and Middle Eastern nations. Spain gained control of the islands in 1521 and ruled them for 377 years, naming them the Philippines after King Philip of Spain. Today, the Spanish cultural influence is still very evident.

The Philippines was ceded to the United States after Spain's defeat in the Spanish-American War. During World War II, when the Japanese were winning the war in the Pacific, the Japanese took over the Philippines. Although, the United States granted independence to the Philippines after the Japanese were defeated in World War II, Americans have a significant social, cultural, and political influence.

The Philippines went through a major political reorganization in 1985 when President Ferdinand Marcos left the country and Corazon Aquino was elected president.

Philippine Culture

As a result of the history of the Philippine Islands, the culture is a mixture of East and West.

The Family

The basic Filipino sociocultural unit is the nuclear family, which includes the father, the mother, and the children. Parents may live with their adult children. The bilaterally extended kinship group includes all the relatives of both the mother and the father, including their cousins. These relatives may live either with the family or in a neighboring house. Thus, the family structure is large.

As a result of this widespread sharing in the kinship circle, individuals tend to be interdependent, relying on the extended family for support and protection. There are family consultations for major decisions. Maintenance of family goodwill is emphasized, and disagreements are kept within the family. Government services for the elderly are minimal because families take care of their elderly members. Many immigrants find it difficult to adjust to the more independent life styles and feel obligated to take care of the elderly.

In the traditional Filipino family, each member has specific roles and responsibilities, both of which are hierarchically defined in the family:

1. Grandparents are accorded the most respect and authority. In the most traditional families, they live with their son's family; the daughter-in-law needs to respect the wishes of her mother-in-law, even in household and child-rearing matters.
2. The father is the nominal head of the family, principal breadwinner, and dispenser of discipline. He has the final say in decisions (although the mother shares in this authority), provides leadership in determining the goals and aspirations of the family, and establishes outside contacts to enhance the family economy.
3. The mother shares in the husband's authority, duties, and responsibilities; assumes responsibility for household management, child-rearing, and religious obligations; and helps augment the family income by obtaining employment or engaging in household industry.
4. Children are the center of family life. Their traditional role is to respect and obey their parents, grandparents, and elders without question. They also have specific duties at home:
   - Older sons share in authority over younger children, assume responsibility for the care and behavior of the younger children, set good examples, and make sacrifices for the care of younger siblings. The eldest assumes the father's role in his absence.
   - Older daughters share in authority over their younger siblings and assume responsibility for routine care, such as dressing, feeding, and ensuring the safety of younger siblings. The eldest assumes the mother's role in her absence.
   - Younger children are expected to listen, obey, and do well by following the examples set by their older siblings. They may be scolded for not following the advice of older siblings.

Each member of a Filipino family must live in a way that brings honor to the ancestors and the family name. In this respect, children are not viewed as individuals who will someday make their own mark in the future. Rather, they are considered another extension of many family generations, the product of that family and ancestry. Problems and successes are shared by the family. Any shortcomings in a family member dishonor the entire family—and the ancestors. This belief is so strong that the handicapped are sometimes ostracized from their family and left on the streets to become beggars.

The roles and responsibilities of the traditional Filipino family may be altered by the impact of immigration, socioeconomic influences in the new societies, and political changes. Even in the Philippines, however, family patterns, practices, and values differ according to the area in which families live (i.e., urban or rural), religious affiliation, ethnic group membership, and socioeconomic status. Like families in other societies that are in the process of modernization, the Filipino family is undergoing changes as a result of population growth, alterations in the roles of men and women, shifting patterns of kin relationships, and other factors. Immigrants from metropolitan areas have been exposed to Eastern and Western cultures, whereas immigrants from rural areas may have a more traditional view.

Cultural Values

The Filipinos place a great value on education. Parents often beg and borrow money, or sell family property, in order to send their children to school. The competition for educational opportunity is fierce, and institutions of higher education cannot admit all the young Filipinos who want to attend. One major motivation for a Filipino family's emigration to the United States is to pursue a better education for the children. According to the State of California Department of Education survey in 1985, there were 37,440 Filipinos enrolled in the California public schools. The number continues to grow as the internal instability of the Philippines causes many families to emigrate. Many go to Hawaii, Guam, and California.

Respect for the old, always strong in Asian countries, is still in evidence in the Philippines. Early in life, Filipino children learn the proper respect for their elders. They learn not to talk unless they are addressed, not to interrupt a conversation, and not to volunteer information. Looking down is considered a sign of respect; conversely, eye contact with elders is viewed as a sign of defiance. Children also learn that they should not even walk in front of an elder. Children must respect the authority and obey the decisions not only of their parents, but also of their teachers and other elders.

A child who falls is not always picked up and coddled. Instead, the child is told to get up without assistance and to behave like an adult. A child who cries after fighting with another child may be told to go back and beat the adversary or to take the beating without a whimper. Should the child cry after that, the child may be punished. Thus, Filipino children are taught that it is cowardly to run away from danger or from an enemy. Child-rearing practices vary from family to family, and therefore, it is difficult to generalize.

Filipinos are sensitive, shy, and quiet. They love to pay compliments, but feel embarrassed when they receive compliments. They tend to avoid direct confrontations or criticisms for fear of hurting the other person's feelings. In the interest of remaining on good terms with people, they tend to agree readily with another's comments, praise them extravagantly, and make remarks that they anticipate will please the listener. In handling delicate matters, such as marriage, money matters, and quarrels, a go-between is usually asked to intervene.

The question of "face" is part of the Oriental character. In an attempt to avoid offending anyone or creating a scene, Filipinos silence their conscience. The outward harmony is valued more highly than "being right." Westerners may regard this as completely outrageous—a voluntary surrender of personal rights. To the Filipino, however, the open expression of emotions is rude and uncultured. Filipinos do not express anger openly, for example. Although they may appear calm and collected, they may be very unhappy and angry. Because of the emphasis on interpersonal relationships and the need for affiliation and cooperation, Filipinos attempt to get along with their companion at all costs in order to maintain self-esteem and social acceptance.

Self-esteem is the preservation of one's dignity in relationship to others. Nothing is considered worse than being shamed. The personal relationship style of Filipinos is markedly different from that of Americans, which may cause some misinterpretation. A favor done for someone must be reciprocated, or it remains a "debt." A person who does not return a favor loses face and may be called shameless.

Hospitality is a prevailing theme in the Philippine culture. A guest is always offered the very best of everything that the family can afford. It is generally considered impolite for the guest to accept food or drink immediately; in order to be polite, the guest must initially refuse the food and drink. The host, however, must insist that the guest have something to eat or drink. The ritual goes back and forth until the guest accepts the offered food or drink. Such styles of communication may be so unusual to Americans that they find them difficult to comprehend.

Filipinos usually rely on family groups and on an "all merciful God" for the solution of individual problems and for the determination of destiny. They prefer to sidestep troublesome issues or problems, leaving them in the hands of God and a deterministic fate. Filipinos seldom worry about the future—if it is their fate to be poor, what can they do? "Utang ng loob" is instilled in the family member, if not, the member is called an "ingrate."

Filipinos derive status primarily from family standing, position, education, and wealth. Rank is accorded importance and deference. Relationships between superior and subordinate are formal; subordinates never call their superior by the first name. In fact, the customs for personal address in social situations are more formal than are those of Americans. Some immigrants find it difficult to adjust to the informal or casual method of address.

Linguistic Background of Filipino Immigrants

The Philippines is a multilingual country. There are 87 mutually unintelligible languages spoken in the country. A person from a northern island cannot understand the language spoken by a person from a southern island. For example, Bicolano is spoken in the south, Pampango is spoken on the main island, Micolum is spoken around the Mindanao area in the south, Pangasinan is spoken in the north, Ilocano is spoken in the mid-Visayan islands, Ilongo is spoken in the west Visayan islands, and Cebuano is spoken in the east Visayan islands. Tagalog is spoken by 60% of the population. (See Figure 4-1.)

The three official languages of the Philippines are Pilipino, English, and Spanish. In 1957, the Philippines National Assembly enacted a law that made Pilipino the national language. This language is based on Tagalog, but it borrows from other Philippine languages.

When the Japanese occupied the Philippines during World War II, the Japanese language was taught in the schools; as a result, some Filipinos know Japanese. Now, English and Pilipino are the medium of instruction, resulting in a bilingual education. Spanish is generally introduced in college. English is the language of formality, while Pilipino is the language for the arts, poetry and literature. Some immigrants from the Philippines speak English and do not

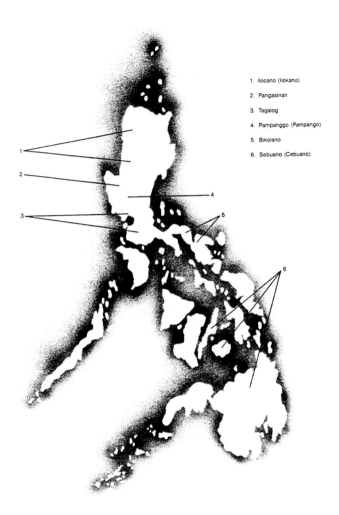

1. Ilocano (Ilokano)
2. Pangasinan
3. Tagalog
4. Pampanggo (Pampango)
5. Bikolano
6. Sebuano (Cebuano)

Figure 4-1 Location of Philippine Language Groups

encounter the difficulty that other Asians encounter when they first arrive in the United States. Many Filipinos speak English with a heavy "accent," however, which may cause some difficulty in communication.

The primary non-English languages spoken within Filipino-American communities in the United States are Pilipino, Ilocano, and Cebuano. Many immigrant children speak more than one Philippine dialect and have learned some English if they were old enough to attend school before they left the Philippines. The extent of their exposure to English and Pilipino outside of school depends on their socioeconomic background and the region of the Philippines in which they lived. The higher the family's socioeconomic status, the more likely that the children have had access to news media, radio, TV programs, and public or private education and, thus, greater exposure to both English and Pilipino. Children who lived in urban areas of the Philippines also have had greater exposure to English and Pilipino through the media.

The Pilipino Language

The Pilipino alphabet has 20 letters: 15 consonants

B K D G H L M N NG P
R S T W Y

and five vowels

A E I O U
a e i o u

In 1976, the Department of Education and Culture of the Philippines modified the orthographic rules of Pilipino in order to accommodate the rapid developments and changes in the Pilipino language brought about by the influx of linguistic elements from different languages, native as well as foreign, and in order to meet the needs of modernization. Because foreign words, particularly proper nouns and words recently introduced into Pilipino may retain their original spelling, the letters *c, ch, f, j, ll, ñ, q, rr, v, x,* and *z* may be used in some cases (Table 4-1). Students are taught to read and write in this system during their first year in school.

Pilipino has 27 phonemes: 16 consonant sounds, including the significant glottal stop; 5 vowel sounds; and 6 diphthongs. Every consonant and vowel sound is represented by one letter in the alphabet, with the exception of the glottal stop ('). Following are the Pilipino consonant sounds under the English consonants that they most closely resemble:

English: b d g l m n ŋ   r v z zh w y th j p t f s sh ch th h
Pilipino: b d g l m n ɲ   r _ _ _ w y _ _ . p t _ s _ _ _ _ h

---

Table 4-1 Loan Words

Foreign Letter	Pilipino Equivalent Letter(s)	Foreign Loan Word	Pilipino Equivalent Word
c	k	calesa	kalesa (horse-driven cart)
ch	ts	chinelas	tsinelas (house slippers)
c	s	circo	sirko (circus)
ch	ts	cha	tsa (tea)
f	p	cafe	cape (coffee)
		fino	pino (fine, texture)
j	h	jota	hota (letter j)
		juez	huwes (judge)
j	s	jabon	sabon (soap)
ll	ly	cepillo	sepilyo (toothbrush)
ll	y	caballo	kabayo (horse)
ñ	ny	niña	ninya (girl)
q	k	tanque	tangke (tank)
		maquina	makina (machine)
rr	r	carro	karo
v	b	virgen	birhen (virgin)
x	ks	taxi	taksi (taxi)
z	s	lapiz	lapis (pencil)
		zapatos	sapatos (shoes)

There are nine consonant sounds in English that do not exist in the Pilipino sound system. Similarly, there are more vowel and diphthong sounds in English than in Pilipino (Table 4-2).

Since there are more sounds in English than in Pilipino, the Pilipino speaker must learn sounds that do not occur in Pilipino in order to understand and be understood in English. For example, the Pilipino speaker must learn to recognize and produce the sounds *f, v, z,* and *th.* A Pilipino speaker tends to substitute *p, b, s,* and *t* for the preceding sounds since they are the most similar sounds that occur in the Pilipino language. For example, the Pilipino speaker might pronounce *fail, vie, measure,* and *thank* as *pail, buy, meashure,* and *tank.*

As mentioned earlier, certain Pilipino sounds cover a wider area than similar sounds in English. For example, the final sound of maram*i* may be said to cover the area that includes roughly the vowel sounds of English *lift* and *left.* Therefore, a Pilipino speaker may have trouble distinguishing, for example, between *lift* and *left.*

Plurality is indicated in most English nominals by *-s;* for example, poem*s,* disk*s,* building*s.* In Pilipino, this idea is expressed by the word *onga* placed before the nominal pluralized (e.g., *onga bata* 'children') or by another word carrying the idea of plural (e.g., *dalawang bata* 'two child' or *maraming bata* 'many child'). Following the Pilipino pattern, the native speaker may say *many friend* instead of *many friends.* He may also overgeneralize the pluralization rule and say *tooths* instead of *teeth.* Some English sounds are sufficiently similar to their Pilipino counterparts that Pilipino speakers have no serious difficulties in learning to pronounce the English sounds. Other English sounds are so dissimilar that, when combined with Pilipino sounds, they result in serious distortions of meanings (Table 4-3).

Pilipino's large-scale borrowings from Spanish and English have resulted in lexical interference of various kinds. One such interference involves the use of

---

Table 4-2 English and Pilipino Vowels and Diphthongs

English		*Pilipino*	
/e/	bed	/e/	eto (here it is)
/i/	meet	/i/	ibn (bird)
/I/	bit		
/ai/	bite	/ay/	kamay (hand)
/ei/	bait	/ey/	reyna (queen)
/æ/	bat		
/u/	but		
/ə/	less<u>o</u>n, bon<u>u</u>s, norm<u>a</u>l		
/ū/	lat<u>er</u>, auth<u>or</u>, sug<u>ar</u>, f<u>ur</u>, f<u>ir</u>, h<u>er</u>		
/o/	hot		
/a/	car, f<u>a</u>ther	/a/	araw (sun, day)
/ô/	or	/o/	oo (yes)
/o/	no		
/u/	pool	/u/	ulo (head)
/U/	pull		
/aw/	now	/aw/	ilaw (light)
/oy/	toy	/oy/	baboy (pig)
		/uy/	aruy (ouch!)
		/iw/	paksiw (a food cooked with vinegar)

Table 4-3 Possible Phonetic Interferences of Pilipino in Learning English

Interference	Sound	Example
Substitution of consonants	b/v	berry/very
	p/f	pour/four
	t/θ	tree/three
	d/ð	dare/there
	ts/tʃ	tseer/cheer
	s/ʃ	sue/shoe
	s/z	sue/zoo
	d/dʒ	duce/juice
	d/ʒ	madder/measure
Deaspiration of aspirated plosive	p/p'	pie
	t/t'	tea
	k/k'	key
Distortion	r/r	river
Substitution of long vowels for short vowels		eat/it
		feet/fit
		fool/full
		coat/caught
		seat/sit
		pool/pull
		odor/order
Confusion	/ɛ/	
	/æ/	
	/a/	
	/ɔ/	
	/e/	
	(e.g., yes, there, sat, set, ox, law)	

false cognates. An incomplete knowledge of the range of meanings often leads the Pilipino speaker to construct sentences that are either amusing or incomprehensible to the native speakers of English and Spanish. For example, the Spanish *destinar* (to destine, appoint, designate, or assign) may be equated with the English *destine* (to predetermine, as by Divine will, or to appoint). Thus, the Pilipino speaker may say, "My father was destined in the province for a year" instead of "My father was assigned to the province for a year."

As noted by Ramos and de Guzman (1971), Pilipino has a complex system of affixation. Most words consist of roots, which are substantive, verbal, and adjectival in meaning, and affixes, which show respect, focus, and mode. The specific meaning of a word is determined by the combination of its root and its affix or affixes. For example, the root *bili* has different meanings, depending on the affix used:

magbili	(verb)	to sell
leumbili	(verb)	to buy
makabili	(verb)	to be able to buy
palabili	(adjective)	fond of buying
bilihin	(noun)	items for sale/to buy

Almost any root in Pilipino may be transformed into a verb by affixation:

dasal	(noun)	prayer
magdasal	(verb)	to pray
tanim	(noun)	plant
magtanim	(verb)	to plant
payag	(adjective)	willing
pumayag	(verb)	to agree

Reduplication is used extensively to show linguistic features such as plurality, intensity, and uncompleted action:

tamad	lazy
matatamad	lazy (plural)
dalawa	two
daladalawa	by twos
dadalawa	only two
dadalawadalawa	the only five (intensification)
laro	to play
maglaro	will play
naglalaro	playing (uncompleted action)

The normal word order for simple sentences in Pilipino is the reverse of that in English; the normal Pilipino word order is

Predicate (or Comment) + Subject (or Topic)

The predicate may be verbal or nonverbal in either language. In Pilipino, however, prepositional phrases and adverbial words may be used as nonverbal predicates. For example,

Verbal Predicate
Natulog ang bata.
Slept the child.

Kumanta ang guro.
Sang the teacher.

Nabili ang baso.
Bought the glass.

Nonverbal Predicate

Nominal	Dentista siya.	
	Dentist he/she.	
Prepositional	Sa San Jose ang parada.	
	In San Jose the parade.	
Adverbial	Bulers ang aksamen.	
	Tomorrow the examination.	

There is, of course, an alternate word order in Pilipino that is similar to the word order in English, but it is used less frequently. Usually, a Pilipino speaker uses this word order to emphasize the first element of the sentence or to make the conversation somewhat more formal:

Normal Word Order	*Alternate Word Order*
Natulog ang bata.	Ang bata ay natulog.
Slept the child.	The child slept.
Dentista siya.	Siya ay dentista.
Dentist he/she.	He/she is a dentist.

As shown in these sentences, there is no equivalent of the verb *to be* in Pilipino. The word *ay* is an inversion marker, not an equivalent of the verb *to be*.

An important feature of Pilipino and other Philippine languages that does not occur in English is termed *focus*. A verbal affix indicates one of the following relationships between the verb and the subject:

1. adjective   Kumain ng mangga ang bata.
   ate a mango the child (agent or actor)
   The child ate a mango.
2. object   Kinain ng bata ang mangga.
   ate the child the mango (object)
   The child ate the mango.
3. locative   Pinagkainan ng bata ang pinggan.
   ate on the child the plate (location)
   The child ate on the plate.

The Pilipino verb system does not make true tense distinctions, but instead characterizes an event as begun or not begun and, if begun, as completed or not completed:

uminom	drank	(begun and completed)
umiiom	drinking	(begun, but not completed)
iinom	will drink	(not begun)

Furthermore, the Pilipino verb is usually not inflected for number; the same form occurs with both singular and plural nouns and pronouns:

Naglalaro siya.	He/she is playing.
Naglalaro sila.	They are playing.

Unlike English, Pilipino does not indicate gender in its third person singular pronouns:

siya	he/she
niy	him/her
kaniya	his/hers

It does, however, distinguish between the first person plural exclusive and inclusive:

kami (exclusive)	tayo (inclusive)	we
namin (exclusive)	natin (inclusive)	our

Pilipino uses linkers or ligatures extensively to connect words, phrases, and sentences that are related to each other as modifiers and modified words. The major linkers are *na* and *-ng*. The linker *na*, which occurs between the modifier and the modified, is used after consonants. The linker *-ng* is attached to the first member of the construction when it ends in a vowel or the letter *n*. When attached to a word ending in *n*, the *n* of *-ng* is dropped. For example:

matalinong mag-aaral	intelligent student
apat na sumbrero	four hats
malakas na ulan	heavy rain
maikling kuwento	short story
magandang bahay	beautiful horse

Clearly, the extent of the phonetic and syntactical differences between Pilipino and English causes many problems for the Pilipino speaker who is learning English.

The Koreans

According to the U.S. Bureau of the Census, there were approximately 700,000 Koreans living in the United States in 1983 (*A Handbook for Teaching Korean Speaking Students*, 1983). Of that number, 130,000 resided in the state of California—approximately 100,000 in the city of Los Angeles. The statistics from the California State Department of Education (*Report on FEP/LEP Students*, 1985) indicate that, in 1985, there were 13,058 Korean students of fluent English proficiency (FEP) and 9,429 Korean students of limited English proficiency (LEP) enrolled in the public schools in the state of California. The total number of Korean-speaking students in California was 22,307, making them the fifth largest group of FEP/LEP students.

Historical Background

Korea was a Chinese colony until 668 A.D., when the Silla Kingdom was formed, unifying all Korean people. The Silla Dynasty was overturned by the Konyo Dynasty (918–1392 A.D.).

In 1910, Japan occupied Korea, and the occupation continued until after World War II. In 1945, the United States and the Soviet Union agreed that the United States would *accept* the surrendered territory south of the 38th parallel and the Soviet Union would *accept* the area north of it, resulting in the formation of North and South Korea. In 1950, North Korea invaded South Korea, and the Korean War began. It lasted 3 years, until the armistice was negotiated in 1953.

Korean immigration to the United States began in the early 1900s when some laborers were brought to Hawaii and later to the mainland. Prior to World War II, however, the Korean community was not very visible because of its small population. The Koreans emigrating to the United States since 1975 have all been from South Korea.

Korean Culture

The Chinese have had a strong influence on Korean culture. In fact, the prevailing themes of Korean culture are similar to those of Chinese culture, namely, harmony, filial piety, reverence for elders, and the importance of social order and family. All the Korean family names are derived from Chinese family names. In addition, most Koreans adhere to the philosophy of Confucianism.

Korean children are often reserved and are taught to control their emotions and behaviors. A well-behaved Korean child generally does not talk back, does not ask many questions, thinks twice before answering a question, and is embarrassed when given attention. They try to excel in school in order to win the approval of their parents.

Koreans believe in social order and adhere to the rules dictating the expected behavior in the five relationships: (1) parents and children, (2) older persons and younger persons, (3) husband and wife, (4) friends, and (5) ruler and subject.

The Korean Language

Koreans in both North and South Korea speak the same language. Although there are some variations among the Korean dialects, they are mutually intelligible. The Korean language belongs to the Altaic language family.

Before 1443 A.D., the Koreans used the Chinese written language. The Korean written language Hangul was created in 1443 A.D., but the Korean family names remained Chinese. The most frequently encountered names are Lee, Chung, Kim, and Park. Although the South Korean government attempted to remove all Chinese characters from the Korean language after World War II, the effort was unsuccessful. At the present time, graduates of Korean high schools are expected to know approximately 1,800 Chinese characters.

The Korean written language has a basic alphabet of 19 consonants (Table 4-4) and 8 vowels (Table 4-5). By combining different consonants (C) and vowels (V), syllables are created. The rules for syllabification allow the following syllabic forms: CV, CVC, CVV, and CVVC. The sound of a letter in a word or a sentence is produced differently according to the position of that letter (Table 4-6).

Because Korean has no consonant clusters in initial or final positions of words, it may be difficult for Korean speakers to produce English consonant clusters. Fricatives and affricates do not occur in the final position in Korean; such consonants may sometimes be omitted by Korean speakers of English. Final stops are often nasalized when they occur before a nasal sound; for example, Korean speakers may say banman for batman; bingham for big man.

Other differences between the phonetic systems of English and Korean create similar difficulties for Korean speakers learning English. Unlike the English vowel system, for example, the Korean system has no contrast in vowel length. Therefore, the following vowels are problematic for Korean speakers: /i/, /I/, /u/, /ʌ/, and /ɔ/.

Table 4-4 Korean Consonants

Manner	Place of Articulation				
	Bilabial	Dental	Palatal	Velar	
Stops	p	t		k	Lax
	b	d		g	Tense
	p'	t'		k	Aspirated
Affricates			c		Lax
			j		Tense
			c'		Aspirated
Fricatives		s		h	Lax
		s:			Tense
Nasals	m	n			
Liquids		l	[r]		

Table 4-5   Korean Vowels

Front	Central		Back	
/i/	/i:/	Unrounded	/µ/	High (close)
/e/	/e:/		/o/	Middle
/æ/	/a/			Low (open)

As there are no labiodental, interdental, or palatal fricatives in Korean, speakers of Korean may make the following substitutions:

b / v
p / v
s / ʃ
s / z
t / tʃ
dz / ð

While there is a three-way contrast in the Korean stops and fricatives (namely, the voiced, the tense voiceless, and lax voiceless), there is only a two-way

Table 4-6   Location of Consonants in Korean Syllable Structure

Korean Letters	Initial	Medial	Final
ㄱ	K	G	K
ㄲ	KK, GG	GG	K
ㅋ	K'	K'	K
ㄴ	N	N	N
ㄷ	T	D	T
ㄸ	TT, DD	DD	
ㅌ	T'	T'	T
ㄹ		R, L	L
ㅁ	M	M	M
ㅂ	P	B	P
ㅃ	PP, BB	BB	P
ㅍ	P'	P'	P
ㅅ	S	S	T
ㅆ	SS	SS	T
ㅈ	CH	J	T
ㅉ	CHCH, JJ	JJ	T
ㅊ	CH'	CH'	T
ㅎ	H	H	T, K
ㅇ		NG	NG

Source: From *First Course in Korean Language* (p. 2) by C. H. Lee, 1965, Seattle: University of Washington Press. Copyright 1965 by University of Washington Press. Reprinted by permission.

contrast in the English stops and fricatives. For example, there are two voiceless ls: labial stops *p, pp*—one is tense and one is lax. The nonaspirated stops and fricatives may be a problem for the Korean speakers.

The /r/ and /l/ sounds in Korean belong to the same phonemic category in allophonic variation. Korean speakers may substitute /r/ for /l/ or vice versa since /l/ occurs in the final position in Korean and /r/ occurs elsewhere in Korean.

Because there is no tonic word stress in Korean, speakers of Korean may sound monotonous when they speak English. They may also find it difficult to formulate wh- questions and tag questions in English such as *isn't it?* and *don't you?* at the end of a question.

Korean has sociolinguistic rules that govern the behavior of individuals in their relationships with others and in particular social contexts. For example, an honorific particle is always attached to an honorable subject, and an honorific infix is inserted in the verb that refers to the honorable subject. The inappropriate use of the particle may be interpreted as an unnecessary formality, and the lack of the particle may be interpreted as disrespect and contempt. Most children acquire the basic rules of honorifics by the age of 6.

In the Korean language, individual words do not change to alter their meaning (e.g., have, had). Instead, the linguistic process of agglutination is used to form lexical items. Their process involves the combination of elements to create compound words or larger linguistic units. For example, a declarative sentence has a declarative sentence ending, and markings carry different semantic meanings. Many other lexical features of Korean differ from those of English:

- There is no gender agreement in the Korean language.
- There are no articles in the Korean language.
- Korean is noninflectional.
- Korean has no relative pronouns.
- Korean verbs are not inflected for tense or number.

Table 4-7 Korean vs. English Syntax

Korean	English
Subject-Object-Verb I water drink	Subject-Object-Verb I drink water
Clause-Conjunction you leave if	Conjunction-Clause if you leave
Noun-Locative Marker house in	Preposition-Noun in the house
Adjective Clause-Noun I bought book	Noun-Adjective Clause The book that I bought
Main Verb-Auxiliary go dare	Auxiliary-Main Verb dare go
Subject-Verb Question Marker? frog jump?	Auxiliary-Subject-Verb? Did the frog jump?
Adverb Phrase-Verb in the morning left	Verb-Adverb Phrase left in the morning

There are also major differences between Korean and English word order (Table 4-7) that cause problems for Koreans who are learning English.

The Japanese

The total land area of Japan is 145,670 square miles, which is approximately 8,000 square miles less than the land area of California. Japan comprises four main islands and more than 500 islets. From north to south, the four large islands are Hokkaido, Honshu, Shikoko, and Kyushu. The terrain is mountainous and volcanic. The population of Japan is 110,000,000, which is approximately 50% of the population of the United States.

Historical Background

Because land in their own country was limited, large numbers of Japanese farmers began to emigrate to the United States (first to Hawaii and then to California) between 1891 and 1907. The census of 1890 reported the number of Japanese residents as 2,039. The number of immigrants increased steadily after that, and the record showed that 10,000 Japanese immigrants entered the United States in 1907. They worked in agriculture, railroad building, mining, and fishing.

There was a change of attitude in California in the early 1900s. The Japanese immigrants encountered hostility and resentment. Large groups of people urged Congress to adopt a resolution to exclude the Japanese totally. In a "Gentlemen's Agreement," Japan pledged to restrict the number of its citizens allowed to emigrate to the United States.

During World War II, the Japanese on the West Coast were sent to internment camps. After World War II, very few Japanese came to the United States. In recent years, however, there has been a steady influx of Japanese immigrants.

Japanese Culture

Chinese culture and Buddhism have influenced Japanese culture heavily. The major themes of Japanese culture are a concern for saving face and the maintenance of harmony. Modesty and humility are regarded as very important virtues. An open display of emotions is considered a sign of weakness.

There is a definite hierarchy in Japanese relationships. Each individual has a defined place in society and a role to play in a myriad of relationships. Furthermore, the individual is expected to accept that place and to play each role well. Unlike the Americans, the Japanese do not consider upward mobility as important as loyalty to their employers. The Japanese success story has intrigued so many researchers that many books have been written about the Japanese style of business management and work ethics.

There are subtle cultural implications in the Japanese communication style. What is said may not be what is meant. It is necessary to read not only all the linguistic signals, but also all the paralinguistic signals in order to determine the semantic meaning of words.

Children are expected to be obedient, respectful, and well-behaved. Elderly people are to be revered. Education is highly valued.

The Japanese Language

Like the Korean language, the Japanese language belongs to the Altaic language family. It was only a spoken language until, in the 8th century, Chinese characters were brought into Japan in the form of Buddhist sutras (writings) and applied to Japanese words. Thus, many characters of the Japanese written system originated in the Chinese written language; these characters are called Kanji.

Although Japanese writing resembles Chinese writing, the Japanese pronunciation of the characters is entirely different from the Chinese pronunciation. Japanese is predominantly polysyllabic and has an elaborate inflectional system. For example, the word *flower* is written as 花 in both Japanese and Chinese, but the Japanese pronounce it hana while the Chinese pronounce it hua. Furthermore, Japanese is not tonal; every syllable in a word is given equal stress. The Japanese modified the Chinese symbols for phonetic purposes, organizing a syllabary called Kana. There are two types of Kana: Katakana and Hiragana. The Katakana is generally used for names and foreign words (Exhibit 4-1). The Hiragana is cursive, used to write Japanese when Chinese characters are not available.

There are a few dialects of Japanese, and the dialectal variations can be great. Someone from Honshu may have difficulty understanding someone from Kyushu. The standard Japanese is taught at school, however, and all official documents, newspapers, and radio and television stations use the standard Japanese.

Japanese has 5 vowels and 18 consonants. The 5 vowels are /a/, /i/, /u/, /e/, and /o/. Like English vowels, Japanese vowels vary in duration. In Hiragana, a long vowel is written in two separate syllables. The vowels /i/ and /u/ are often not pronounced when they appear between voiceless consonants, such as /f/, /h/, /k/, /p/, /s/, /t/, /sh/, and /ch/. The 18 Japanese consonants are /k/, /s/, /t/, /n/, /h/, /m/, /y/, /r/, /w/, /g/, /d/, /b/, /z/, /p/, /ch/, /sh/, /ts/, and /j/. Double consonants, such as /kk/ and /pp/, may occur. Only the /n/ phoneme may occur as a final consonant in Japanese. The phonetic system of their native language may interfere with the learning process of Japanese who are trying to learn English (Table 4-8).

Salient grammatical features of the Japanese language include the following:

- The prefix *o* is used as a term for politeness rather than as a part of a word. For example, sushi is a common food, but osushi is a more polite way of saying the same word.
- The suffix *san* is also used as a term of politeness. For example, untenshu means driver, but untenshu-san means Mr. Driver.
- All verbs appear in the final position of the sentence.
- Personal pronouns are often omitted, since they are inferred from the context.
- Nominal markers and particles are used to indicate locations, directions, or grammatical functions. Markers and particles serve different grammatical functions. Markers are used to change the meaning of an utterance, e.g., positive to negative. Particles are used to convey social meanings such as honorific status or a question.

Kore wa hon desu.

This *marker topic* book

Exhibit 4-1 The Japanese Language

THE KA-TA-KA-NA SYLLABARY
(formed in 8th Century)

	A ア	I イ	U ウ	E エ	O オ
K	KA カ	KI キ	KU ク	KE ケ	KO コ
S	SA サ	SHI シ	SU ス	SE セ	SO ソ
T	TA タ	CHI チ	TSU ツ	TE テ	TO ト
N	NA ナ	NI ニ	NU ヌ	NE ネ	NO ノ
H	HA ハ	HI ヒ	FU フ	HE ヘ	HO ホ
M	MA マ	MI ミ	MU ム	ME メ	MO モ
Y	YA ヤ	I イ	YU ユ	E エ	YO ヨ
R	RA ラ	RI リ	RU ル	RE レ	RO ロ
W	WA ワ	I ヰ	U ウ	E ヱ	O ヲ
	-NG ン				

SONANT & HALF-SONANT SYLLABLES

	A	I	U	E	O
G	GA ガ	GI ギ	GU グ	GE ゲ	GO ゴ
Z	ZA ザ	JI ジ	ZU ズ	ZE ゼ	ZO ゾ
D	DA ダ			DE デ	DO ド
B	BA バ	BI ビ	BU ブ	BE ベ	BO ボ
P	PA パ	PI ピ	PU プ	PE ペ	PO ポ

Source: From *Instant Japanese* (p. 28) by M. Watanabe and K. Nagashima, 1964, Tokyo, Japan: Yohan Publications, Inc. Copyright 1964 by Yohan Publications, Inc. Reprinted by permission.

- There is no distinction between the singular and the plural. For example, hon means book and books.
- Because yes/no questions are marked by a final particle, question markers may not be needed at the initial position of the sentence. A question marker is generally used at the initial position of a sentence, however.
- When a negative form is used in a question, such as ''Don't you want to go?'' the answer ''yes'' means ''yes, you are right. I don't want to go.''
- Relative clauses precede the nouns (in contrast to English, where relative clauses follow nouns).
- Particles are used at the end of sentences to perform various semantic and pragmatic functions.

There are close to 100 ways of saying I or me in Japanese (Exhibit 4-2). The word *I* is different for men and women, young and old, city folk and country folk. It varies according to the pragmatic contexts, such as among friends, with

Table 4-8 Possible Phonetic Interferences of Japanese in Learning English

Interference	Sound	Example
Substitution	r/l	fright/flight
		rice/lice
		right/light
	s/th	sank/thank
		sum/thumb
		sink/think
	z/th	zat/that
	j/th	jis/this
	b/v	belly/very
		bine/vine
Additions of vowel to words ending in a consonant		desker/desk
		milku/milk
		hoteru/hotel
		beddu/bed
Approximation	/f/ phoneme between /f/ and /h/ phonemes	four/whore food/hood

superiors, or at business meetings. Special words are used for I in correspondence.

The People of the Hawaiian Islands

Mark Twain once called the Hawaiian islands the "loveliest fleet of islands anchored in any sea." The state of Hawaii comprises several main islands: Hawaii, Oahu, Maui, Kauai, Molokai, and Lanai. Kauai is the oldest of the islands and Hawaii is the largest (Figure 4-2). These islands form a 1,500-mile archipelago. The state's main industries are tourism, sugar, and pineapples. The islands are known for their tropical rain forests and waterfalls. There is a vast array of tropical flowers, fruits, and plants, including many species of palms, bromeliads, gingers, heliconias, exotic ornamentals, plants of medicinal value, as well as rare and endangered species.

The islands are multiethnic and multicultural. The main ethnic groups are Japanese, Caucasian, Filipino, Chinese, and Korean. Many languages are spoken in Hawaii, including Hawaiian, Japanese, Mandarin, Cantonese, Korean, Tagalog, Ilocano, Cebuano, Visayan, Pampango, Samoan, Vietnamese, Laotian, Khmer, Thai, Marshallese, Palauan, Chamorro, Pangasinan, Fijian, Spanish, and Portugese. Many words in the Hawaiian language are used by the local people, such as aloha (hello or goodbye); mahalo (thank you); pau (finish); dakine (all); kai (water); mauka (toward the mountain); and makai (toward the ocean). The local people also share many customs of the Polynesian culture, the most famous of which is the luau, the traditional Hawaiian feast.

In a recent publication, Kanehele (1986) noted that the most important Hawaiian values include "aloha," generosity, graciousness, spirituality, friendliness, hospitality, cleanliness, intelligence, and competitiveness. The extended family

Exhibit 4-2 List of I's in Japanese

1. A	33. Ka-jin	63. Sō
2. A-i	34. Ken-ge	64. So-re-ga-
3. A-ko	35. Ko-chi	65. shi
4. A-re	36. Ko-chi-to	65. Te-ma-e
5. A-shi	37. Ko-chi-to-	66. Tō-hō
6. As-shi	ra	67. Tō-sho-ku
7. A-ta-i	38. Kō-do	68. U-chi
8. A-ta-ki	39. Ko-ko-	69. U-ra
9. A-ta-ku-	mo-to	70. U-se-i
shi	40. Ko-na-ta	71. U-se-tsu
10. A-ta-shi	41. Ma-ro	72. Wa
11. A-te	42. Mi	73. Wa-chi-ki
12. Bo-ku	43. Mi-do-mo	74. Wa-ga-ha-
13. Chin	44. Mi-zu-ka-	i
14. Da-i-kō	ra	75. Wa-ga-mi
15. Da-ra	45. Na-ni-ga-	76. Wa-i
16. Fu-bin	shi	77. Wa-ki
17. Fu-ko-ku	46. O	78. Wa-na-mi
18. Fu-shō	47. O-i-don	79. Wan-de-ra
19. Ge-kan	48. O-i-ra	80. Wa-ra-wa
20. Ge-se-tsu	49. O-no	81. Wa-re
21. Ge-shō	50. O-no-re	82. Wa-shi
22. Gi-ra	51. O-ra	83. Wa-ta-i
23. Go-jin	52. O-re	84. Wa-ta-ku-
24. Gu	53. O-re-ra	shi
25. Gu-se-i	54. O-ta-ki	85. Wa-ta-shi
26. Gu-sō	55. Ra	86. Wa-te
27. Hi-shō	56. Ses-sha	87. Ya-ra
28. Hon-kan	57. Se-tsu	88. Ya-se-i
29. Hon-sho-	58. Shō	89. Ya-se-tsu
ku	59. Shō-kan	90. Ya-tsu-ga-
30. I-gi	60. Shō-se-i	re
31. In	61. Shō-shi	91. Yo
32. Ji-bun	62. Shō-te-i	92. Yo-ha-i
		93. Yo-no-mon

Source: From *Instant Japanese* (pp. 145–146) by M. Watanabe and K. Nagashima, 1964, Tokyo, Japan: Yohan Publications, Inc. Copyright 1964 by Yohan Publications, Inc. Reprinted by permission.

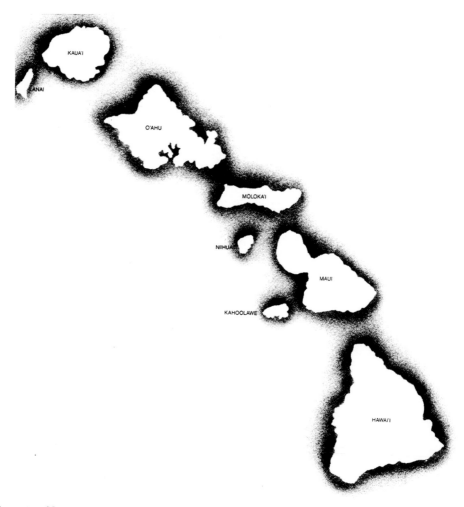

Figure 4-2   Hawaiian Islands

"ohana" is highly valued. The Hawaiian sense of time is expressed best by the statement "you get there when you get there."

The Hawaiian language is polysyllabic and alphabetical (although it has the shortest alphabet in the world). There are five vowels, ā, ē, ī, ō, ū and eight consonants, h, k, l, m, n, p, w, and a glottal stop ?. The consonants are produced the same as they are in English with the exception of w. When w follows an i or e, it is usually produced as v; when it is the first letter of the word or follows an a, there is no rule and pronunciation follows custom. The basic rules are (1) the stress is placed on the second to the last syllable, (2) there are no consonant clusters, (3) the final phoneme is always a vowel, and (4) glottal stop is used (e.g., kou means you and k'ou means mine). Many Hawaiian words are composed of more than two vowels, such as heiau (ancient places of worship). Plantation Pidgin is also spoken by some local residents. Sentences such as "You go stay go" (you go first) and "I go stay come" (I go later) are common phrases.

The Hawaiian language has many loan words from English. The following is a list of some examples:

Hawaiian	English
waina	wine
laki	lucky
kini	king
Iesus	Jesus
kikiki	ticket
kaimana	diamond
hipa	sheep

The Hawaiian vowels are front unrounded (/i/, /e/, and /a/) and back rounded (/u/, and /o/). The stressed vowels are slightly longer than the unstressed vowels. There are two types of vowel combinations: diphthong (such as <u>ai</u>na when the stress falls on the first vowel) and cluster (such as i<u>a</u>le). The length of the vowels changes the meaning of words. For example:

kanaka	man	nana	to plait
kānaka	men	nāna	by him
mala	ache	hio	to blow
māla	whole	hiō	to learn

Both /p/ and /k/ are voiceless stops in Hawaiian consonants. The glottal stop is the second most common consonant in Hawaiian. The following is a list of examples of minimal pairs:

ala	road	'ala	fragrant
kai	ocean	ka'i	to lead
kiki	to sting	ki'i	picture

The /h/, /l/, /m/, and /n/ are pronounced in a way that is similar to the pronunciation of English phonemes. The consonant /w/ has an alternate. The following is a guide for pronunciation (Elbert & Pukui, 1985):

Pronunciation	Spelling
/iv-/	iwa (nine)
/-ev-/	'Ewa (place name)
/-uw-/	auwa'i (ditch)
/-ow-/	'owai (who)
/-aw-, av-/	'awa (a plant)
/w-, v-,/	wahine (woman)

In Hawaii, the LEP population is referred to as the SLEP population (student with limited English proficiency). The 1986 statistics from the Honolulu school district indicated that a total of 8,933 SLEP students speaking more than 22 languages are enrolled in the school district.

The People of Guam and the Micronesian Islands

A territory of the United States, Guam lies at the southern end of the Mariana Islands in the western Pacific; it is the largest island in the Pacific Ocean between

Hawaii and the Philippines. Guam is nearly 30 miles long and 4 to 9 miles wide. The island is volcanic in origin and covers an area of approximately 212 square miles.

The official languages of Guam are English and Chamorro. Both languages are taught in the public and private schools and appear in official documents. The current population of Guam is estimated to be approximately 116,000. Chamorros make up the largest ethnic group, representing approximately 42% of the total population. Caucasians account for approximately 24%; Filipinos, approximately 21%. Other ethnic groups include the Japanese, the Koreans, the Chinese, and those from other Pacific islands.

The Republic of Palau is situated at the western end of the Pacific Islands. The Commonwealth of the Northern Mariana Islands and the Federated States of Micronesia lie in the middle, and the Republic of the Marshall Islands comprises the southernmost group of islands. There are more than 2,200 islands and islets in this general area. The big islands include Palau, Yap, Truk, Pohnpei, and Kosrae. There are seven historical culture groups: Palauans, Southwest Islanders, Mariana Islanders, Yapese, Central Carolinians, Eastern Carolinians, and Marshallese; the eight languages spoken by these islanders are Palauan, Yapese, Trukese, Pohnpeian, Kosraean, Chamorro, Polynesian, and Marshallese.

Historical Background

The Chamorros are believed to have migrated to Guam as early as 2000 B.C. Linguistic and archaeological evidence suggests that they probably came from Indonesia and the Philippines. Ferdinand Magellan sailed into Umatac Bay in 1521, and Spanish missionaries, soldiers, and government officials followed in the 1600s; Guam became a colony of Spain. The Spaniards left an enduring legacy in the religion, culture, architecture, family names, and language of the Chamorros. In 1898, when the United States defeated Spain in the Spanish-American war, Guam was under the administration of the U.S. Department of the Navy. The Japanese occupied Guam for 2½ years during World War II, but the United States regained control after the war.

Germany bought all the islands of Micronesia in 1899, but the League of Nations mandated the transfer of control of the Northern Marianas to Japan in 1920. Japan was in control until World War II; then the U.S. Department of the Navy managed the Northern Marianas until 1962, when their administration was transferred by an act of the United Nations to the United States Trust Territory.

Micronesian Culture

The Chamorro culture places a great deal of emphasis on family and festivities. Celebrations in honor of the patron saints of the island's 19 villages highlight Guam's weekend social life. These fiestas focus on food, such as roast pig, fish, taro, coconut, breadfruit, and sometimes fruit bat. The Guamanian customs and beliefs are similar to those of other Micronesians.

Although there are political and linguistic differences among the Islanders, and although some islands are separated by thousands of miles of the Western Pacific, Micronesians share many customs, beliefs, superstitions, and proverbs.

The theme of the sea permeates their folktales, proverbs, and superstitions. Their legends are part of a rich heritage of oral literature. In these legends, magic often prevails. In general, Micronesians are willing to believe in the legends and myths. Their narratives focus on important aspects of Micronesian culture, frequently communicating a set of values; proverbs are spoken widely to provide lessons in life for adults and children alike.

The weather is warm throughout the year and there is sufficient rainfall. The primary staple foods grown in the Pacific Islands are breadfruit, taro, yams, pandanis, cassava, sweet potatoes, and arrowroot. The most plentiful fruit is coconut; its meat is used for food and its liquid for drinks. In addition, oil can be produced from the coconut for cooking. Fish and pork are the most common main dishes, but dogs, chickens, and fruit bats are also eaten. When visitors arrive at a home, they are served food immediately. The spirit of sharing whatever is available dominates the Micronesian household.

The skills valued in Micronesian cultures are fishing, carpentry, and farming. These skills are taught within extended families and clans. The atolls of Micronesia are generally not conducive to farming, and the people there are more skilled in fishing. The highlanders, such as the Yapese, Pohnpeians, and Kosraens, are more skilled in agriculture. Because the skill of healing is kept as a family secret and passed down from generation to generation, little is known about native medical techniques.

Relatively few people practice polygamy in Micronesia, and all societies in Micronesia are exogamous. The society is matriarchal, and some marriages are still arranged. Wedding ceremonies generally take place at a Catholic or Protestant church. Traditionally, the couple resides with the husband's family. In recent years, there has been an increase in the number of marriages between Micronesians and non-Micronesians.

The birth of a child is the most important occasion in island life. Today, childbirth in Micronesia blends modern medical practice with traditional spiritualism and medicines. Many restrictions are placed on a woman both during pregnancy and immediately after delivery. It is also common for Micronesian children to be adopted, usually through a verbal agreement during the child's first year. Children are born into a number of traditional social structures, including their own family, the nuclear family, the clan, and a political division (i.e., their former tribe).

The death of an island community member is strongly felt. Friends and relatives flock to the home of the deceased as soon as they hear the news. The mourning continues through the night, and a local religious choir sings for the family. With the coming of dawn, visitors return to their homes to gather foods for the feast after the burial. One year after the death, an announcement appears in the newspaper, and a final feast is held in the home of the deceased. Fatalism about death is a prevailing theme in Micronesian culture.

The Chamorro Language

There are 6 vowels in Chamorro (Table 4-9). There are at least 11 vowel allophones of these 6 phonemic vowels (Table 4-10). There are 18 consonants and 1 semiconsonant /w/ in Chamorro. Table 4-11 illustrates the approximate English equivalents of the Chamorro consonants; Table 4-12 is a phonemic consonant chart.

Table 4-9 Phonemic Vowel Chart of Chamorro

	Front	Back
High	i /hita/	u /uchan/
Middle	e /épanglao/	o /oppe/
Low	æ /bæba/	a /baba/

Table 4-10 Phonetic Vowel Chart of Chamorro

	Front	Central	Back
High	i		u
Lower High	ɪ		ʊ
Middle	e	ə	o
Lower Middle	ɛ		ɔ
Low		æ a	

Source: From *Chamorro Reference Grammar* (p. 23) by D. M. Topping, 1973, Honolulu, Hawaii: University Press of Hawaii. Copyright 1973 by University Press of Hawaii. Reprinted by permission.

Table 4-11 Approximate English Equivalents of Chamorro Consonants

Chamorro Consonant	Approximate English Equivalent
/p/	pat
/t/	tap
/k/	king
/b/	bat
/d/	dock
/g/	get
/ch/	tsar
/y/	floods
/f/	fast
/s/	say
/h/	hot
/m/	mama
/n/	not
/ñ/	canyon
/ng/	singing
/l/	long
/r/	rat
/w/	Gwendolyn

Source: From *Chamorro Reference Grammar* (p. 27) by D. M. Topping, 1973, Honolulu, Hawaii: University Press of Hawaii. Copyright 1973 by University Press of Hawaii. Reprinted by permission.

Table 4-12 Phonemic Consonant Chart of Chamorro

	Bilabial	Labiodental	Alveolar	Palatal	Velar	Glottal
Stops						
Voiceless	p		t		k	
Voiced	b		d		g	
Affricates						
Voiceless			ch			
Voiced			y			
Fricatives		f	s			h
Nasals	m		n	n	ng	
Liquids			l,r			
Semiconsonant	w					

Source: From *Chamorro Reference Grammar* (p. 27) by D. M. Topping, 1973, Honolulu, Hawaii: University Press of Hawaii. Copyright 1973 by University Press of Hawaii. Reprinted by permission.

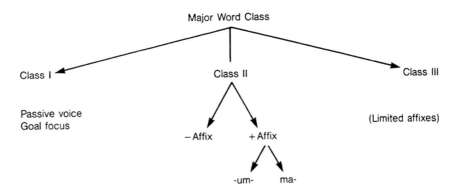

Figure 4-3 Classes of Words in Chamorro

There are three classes of words in Chamorro (Figure 4-3). Class I words must be able to take the passive voice prefix *ma-* and to form the predicate of a goal-focused construction. Class II words can form the predicate of a sentence with the pronoun *yo'* as the subject pronoun. Class III words are subclassed into a, b, c, and d groups because they require different grammatical structures.

There are four basic sentence types in Chamorro: (1) transitive, (2) intransitive, (3) stative, and (4) existential. A basic transitive sentence can be transformed into the others. Intransitive sentences are structured as verb + subject. Stative sentences are constructed in the predicate + subject word order. An existential sentence is composed of a group of irregular verbs.

Like other Asians, those who speak Chamorro are likely to have unique problems in learning English because of the particular characteristics of their native language.

Conclusion

Although the history of the current Filipino, Korean, Japanese, Hawaiian, Guamanian, and Micronesian immigrants to the United States differs from that of the current Indochinese immigrants, these groups share many cultural values. Furthermore, like all immigrants, they have a common need to master the language of their host country. For this, they may need the services of a speech-language-hearing specialist.

PART II

Language Services to Asian Language Minority Populations: The Crisis

CHAPTER 5

Barriers to Language Services

Never in history have more language minorities lived in the United States. The influx of the refugees from Vietnam, Cambodia, and Laos in the 1970s, as well as the immigrants from China, Taiwan, and Hong Kong in the early 1980s, changed the immigration profile significantly, rapidly making the United States more linguistically and culturally diverse. There are more language minority students enrolled in the public schools now than at any other time in U.S. history.

In 1979, there were 7,426 Vietnamese students of limited English proficiency (LEP) in California (California State Department of Education). Their number increased to 14,018 in 1980, to 22,826 in 1981. Thus, there was an increase of 88.8% between 1979 and 1980, an increase of 62.8% between 1980 and 1981. The total number of Asian language minority LEP students in California increased from approximately 36,000 in 1979 to approximately 66,000 in 1981.

In 1981, in the state of California, 18% of the 376,794 pupils who had a limited or no ability to speak English had a Vietnamese, Cantonese, Korean, Pilipino/Tagalog, Portuguese, Mandarin, Japanese, Cambodian, or Laotian language background. In 1983, of the 457,542 identified LEP pupils, more than 120,000, or 26% were native speakers of Vietnamese, Cantonese, Korean, Pilipino, Mandarin, Japanese, Portuguese, Ilocano, Punjabi, Armenian, Laotian, Cambodian, or Samoan (California State Census, 1983). The dramatic increase in the number of immigrants from Asia between 1979 and 1983 is reflected in the fact that the number of Vietnamese LEP students increased from 7,426 in 1979 to 29,037 in 1983—a 29% increase. Furthermore, the number of Cantonese-speaking LEP students increased from 7,219 in 1979 to 15,870 in 1983—a 120% increase.

In the spring of 1985, there were 524,082 LEP students and 503,695 students with fluent English proficiency (FEP) in California. Table 5-1 provides the state summary of LEP/FEP students whose first language is one of seven major Asian languages. Figure 5-1 shows the growth in the number of LEP students in California's public schools from 1973 to 1984. There are similarly large pockets (populations) of Indochinese refugees in various other states, such as Texas, Florida, and New York (Table 5-2).

According to the 1980 census, 34.5 million (15%) of the U.S. population is composed of native speakers of various minority languages (ASHA 1985 Directory of

Table 5-1 Enrollment of Asian Students with Limited English Proficiency (LEP) and Fluent English Proficiency (FEP) in California Public Schools—1985

Languages	LEP Students	FEP Students
Vietnamese	29,990	17,227
Cantonese	19,118	15,669
Korean	9,249	13,058
Pilipino	12,145	25,295
Mandarin	7,009	6,388
Japanese	3,679	6,450
Cambodian	10,730	2,005
Laotian	8,869	1,631
Total	100,789	87,723
Total Asian LEP/FEP Students		188,512

Source: Data from California State Department of Education Bilingual Office.

Bilingual Professionals.) The American Speech-Language-Hearing Association (ASHA) has estimated that at least 3.5 million of these speakers have a speech, language, or hearing disorder that is unrelated to their foreign language use. Thus, the rapid growth of Asian minority populations poses significant challenges to language and local education agencies. For speech, language, and hearing professionals, the challenges are even more demanding. They must deal not only with the school-aged and the preschool population, but also with adults who have communication disorders; they must provide not only habilitative services, but also rehabilitative services. In order to meet the needs of these underserved language minority populations, a multifaceted plan of service delivery is necessary.

Based on the historical, cultural, and linguistic backgrounds of the Asian language minority populations, it is clear that the provision of services to these groups is a complex process that requires multilevel planning and coordination. Furthermore, there are some critical barriers that must be overcome. Some of the general barriers that relate to the delivery of speech, language, and hearing services to the Asian language minorities include the limited number of trained professionals, the lack of available training programs, and the need for all professionals to acquire cross-cultural communication competence. These barriers are not isolated; to the contrary, each has an impact on the others, increasing the complexity of the problems.

Institutional Barriers

Some institutional policies discourage minority students from applying for admission to undergraduate or graduate training programs in speech-language pathology and audiology. New immigrants, refugees, or foreign students do not generally do well on the Graduate Record Examination or the Test of English as a Foreign Language (TOEFL) and, thus, may not qualify for training programs. Consequently, it is difficult to recruit students from Asian language minority backgrounds for these programs.

Training programs require high-level academic skills, which often means an "excellent institutional command" of the English language. First-generation immigrants in such programs may still be struggling with the English language, however, and may find it difficult to survive in such competitive fields as the study of speech and hearing. Policies discourage those who speak with a foreign accent from

LIMITED ENGLISH PROFICIENT STUDENTS (thousands)
525
500
475
450
425
400
375
350
325
300
275
250
225
200
175
525,000 (est.)
+7%
487,835
457,542
+6%
431,443
+15%
376,794
+16%
325,748
+13%
290,082 (a)
288,427
-20%
+24%
+24%
233,520
233,444 (b)
+24%
188,159
1972
73
74
75
76
77*
78
79
80
81
82
83
84
85
YEAR

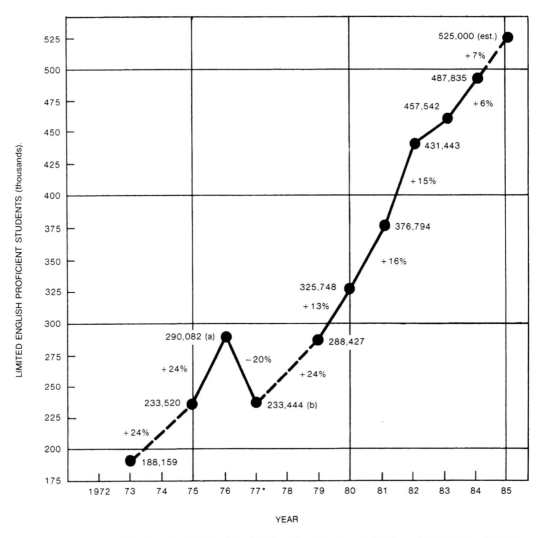

Figure 5-1 The Growth of Limited English Proficient Students in California's Public Schools, 1973 to 1984

Source: California State Department of Education, Office of Bilingual Bicultural Education.

Table 5-2 Enrollment of Asian Students with Limited English Proficiency (LEP) in New York Public Schools

	LEP Students	
Languages	*1983–1984*	*1981–1982*
Vietnamese	2,088	1,902
Chinese	8,539	5,836
Korean	2,016	1,614
Cambodian (Khmer)	922	582
Japanese	978	854
Laotian	639	720
Pilipino	155	183

Source: Data from California State Department of Education Bilingual Office.

participating fully in their clinical training program. The students are penalized because they lack practice in academic English and may not do well in examinations. They may be unable to meet the grade point average requirements set up by the institution. Because it takes many years for adult immigrants and refugees to learn English as a second language and because they usually have difficulty reaching nativelike fluency and literacy, it is extremely difficult for them to cope with a heavy academic load. So far, only a handful of Asian immigrants have graduated from the speech and hearing training programs in the United States.

Instructional Barriers

Traditionally, most Asian schooling is restrictive and rigid. Students learn by memorizing materials from lectures and books, and teachers' questions are generally designed to elicit facts rather than to provoke original thought. Asian students lack the study skills required to do research; to write a position paper, a critique, or a summary; or to propose a topic for a project. In fact, the idea of working on an original project is uncommon in most Asian educational institutions.

It is difficult for instructors to determine how much of the material an Asian student actually understands. Superficially, Asian students may appear to understand lectures. Few of them ask questions, even when asked whether they have questions. Many go home and try to look up in the dictionary vocabulary and/or concepts that they did not understand, but fail to find them. This leads to a sense of frustration and inadequacy. Many of those who begin a training program in the study of speech and hearing drop out after the first semester. Those who continue in spite of the struggle often experience tremendous pressure and anxiety because of their lack of training in academic skills (e.g., writing research papers). Most Asian language minority students feel that the instructors speak too fast, use "big words," and are difficult to follow.

The study habits of Asian students are markedly different from those of Americans in that Asians read word by word and page by page, often failing to integrate, organize, and synthesize the information that they have. They read laboriously and write awkwardly. The manner in which Asian students express thoughts in their native language compounds their problems in reading and writing English. For example, Chinese speakers find it particularly difficult to deal with counterfactual, hypothetical material (Bloom, 1973).

Chen (1985) illustrated the difficulties of Asian students in writing English by means of two passages with the same meaning (Exhibit 5-1). Furthermore, Chen analyzed the two passages syntactically and concluded that the first passage is organized in a coordinated manner, that is, the context is organized in a nonlinear way, and the second in a linear fashion, which makes it far easier to read.

In general, professors do not have a comprehensive understanding of the cultural factors that influence the Asian language minority students' behavior in the classroom. Professors may be unaware of differences in Asian learning styles and communication skills that affect the Asian students' willingness to interrupt, comment, volunteer information, ask questions, and answer questions. Professors may also be unaware of the kinds of difficulties that these students are experiencing.

As a result of their lack of understanding, professors may perceive the students as "quiet," "shy," "passive," or "unresponsive." Furthermore, professors expect the same quality of work from all students and may not be willing to adjust their requirements to meet the needs of the individual students. Undoubtedly, the Asian

Exhibit 5-1 Nonlinear vs. Linear Written Expression

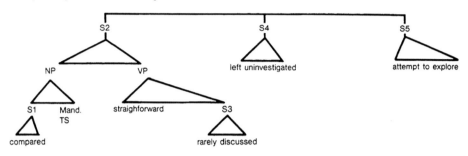

1. Compared to some other Chinese dialects, tone sandhi phenomena in Mandarin are so straightforward that they have rarely been discussed in detail, thus many problems have been left uninvestigated. This paper is an attempt to explore some of those problems.

Note: NP = Noun Phrase   S2 = Sentence 2
VP = Verb Phrase   S3 = Sentence 3
TS = Tone Sandhi   S4 = Sentence 4
S1 = Sentence 1   S5 = Sentence 5

2. This paper is an attempt to explore some of the neglected problems concerning Mandarin tone sandhi phenomena, which have been rarely discussed in detail because they appear to be straightforward in comparison to other dialects.

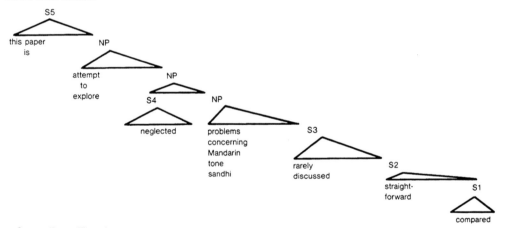

Source: From *Three Representations of Two Semantically Equivalent Paragraphs,* an unpublished presentation, by M. Chen, 1985.

language minority students will not have the English skills of their fellow students at first. They need more time and experience to nurture their English skills. At the same time, they need special attention and assistance from their instructors so that they can overcome linguistic, psychological, and academic barriers.

Legal and Political Barriers

The decisions of U.S. political leaders determine federal and state legislation that affects the lives of all citizens. Changes in immigration laws may increase the number of immigrants and, thus, the number of individuals who require speech, language, or hearing services. The *Lau v. Nichols* (1974) mandate clearly changed special education services and paved the way for bilingual services. In this landmark case, the U.S. Supreme Court ruled unanimously in favor of the plaintiffs from San Francisco's Chinatown. The Court asserted that the equal rights provisions of the U.S. Constitution prohibited withholding from these Chinese the means of comprehending the language of instruction. The plaintiffs held that equal rights in education meant more than equivalent facilities and materials, but also included the language of instruction. This and other similar cases led to the passage of the Bilingual Education Act of 1976. Public Law 95-561 mandates bilingual speech, language, or hearing services for bilingual children. It is clear that government policies affect the services delivered to language minority populations.

The success of equal employment opportunity policies should be evaluated. In general, employers expect their prospective employees to be proficient in English, and Asian language minority speakers may not stand an equal chance in employment because they do not possess "perfect" command of the English language.

Psychosocial Barriers

First-generation immigrants often feel that they do not have sufficient skills in English to pursue a career as a clinician in speech and hearing. They are intimidated when supervisors ask them to undergo "speech therapy" themselves because they speak with a "foreign accent" or ask them not to work with certain types of clients because they do not speak "standard English." Sometimes, clients request a change of clinicians because the clinician assigned to them speaks with a foreign accent. Such occurrences decrease the self-esteem and self-confidence of Asian language minority students who want to become clinicians. The psychological pressures are great; therefore, many Asian individuals who are proficient in their native languages and would be likely candidates for careers as language therapists for Asian LEP students never even enroll in training programs.

Second- or third-generation children of immigrants may become proficient in English and find their proficiency "prestigious." Preferring to use English, they gradually lose the ability to communicate bilingually. Some of the second-generation Asians spoke their native language before they went to school, but gradually lost their ability to speak their native language as they spent more time at school and away from home. Some maintain partial competency in their native language, but require extensive training before they are proficient bilinguals. Others are not able to function in their home language and will not be able to gain fluency unless they take courses in their home language.

Although most Asian families maintain a strong sense of heritage and family ties, some families are assimilated into the mainstream culture and retain very little of their ethnic and cultural tradition. The second and third generations of such families may have little understanding of their native culture. In other words, individuals do not automatically become culturally sensitive because they come from a particular ethnic or racial group. On the other hand, individuals can become bicultural and multicultural if they have had enough exposure, experience, and understanding of those cultures.

Some Asian language minority young people experience marginality, cultural shock, and confusion, resulting in such behaviors as alcohol abuse, participation in organized gangs, and fighting. They have a poor self-image and do not function well. Obviously, people who have problems coping with daily life are seldom motivated to continue their education. Furthermore, many have financial difficulties and cannot afford to go to school.

Those minority students who do continue their education may find it necessary to work 10, 20, or more hours a week to meet their educational expenses. A recent survey from the University of California at Berkeley (Wong-Filmore, 1983) indicates that Asian students work an average of 27 hours per week. This presents special problems, as these students need extra time to increase their proficiency in English and to improve their academic skills. Moreover, these students take longer to complete their assignments than do American students.

Equal educational opportunity policies should be studied to ensure the availability of scholarships, assistantships, and fellowships to the Asian language minority individuals. Policies regarding scholarships and financial aid for immigrant students, as well as government loans for these students, should be examined.

Educational Training Barriers

There are few programs that train individuals to provide speech, language, and hearing services to multicultural populations. Coursework in skill assessment and intervention for bilingual multicultural populations is largely nonexistent, and programs do not provide practicum opportunities for working with these populations. Thus, there is a lack of speech-language pathologists and audiologists in the schools, hospitals, and clinics where language minority populations receive services.

Currently there is a lack of professionals qualified to train potential professionals to work with Asian language minorities. This situation creates a vicious cycle; the lack of trainers creates a lack of trainees, and the lack of trainees creates a lack of potential trainers.

Information Resource Barriers

Professional information about the Asian language minority populations—their languages, cultures, and ways of life—is limited. Furthermore, there are few resources on the development and acquisition of Asian languages, or on Asians' acquisition of a second language, such as intervention materials, English as a second language (ESL) test instruments, and research data. Thus, many of the professionals who have been working with the Asian language minorities have developed their own materials and test instruments. There is a need for networking among the few professionals who work in this field so that they can share information, materials, resources, and insights.

The fact that training institutions do not generally offer courses in multiculturalism and bilingualism contributes to their graduates' lack of information about the current status of the multicultural populations. Because training programs fail to develop and promote cultural pluralism in speech, language, and hearing clinicians, monolingual English-speaking professionals are rarely prepared to work with culturally diverse populations. Even so, clinicians are required to provide some services to multicultural populations. Many clinicians seek assistance from community agencies, bilingual aides, or bilingual interpreters; others just try to handle their caseload with what they know are insufficient and inadequate services.

In addition, the Asian language minority population may not be informed of the services available to them. Most seek help first from physicians who speak their language. Physicians may not have information regarding available speech and hearing services, however. Most Asian parents are unfamiliar with the educational system and are reluctant to participate in parent conferences. They find meetings with school personnel such as IEP conferences overwhelming and sometimes cannot comprehend this and other facets of the education process. They prefer to leave education and remediation to the specialists. Asian clients may not be aware of the rehabilitation services available to them because they do not understand explanations given to them in the English language.

Cultural Barriers

Some Asian family members may feel that there is nothing that can be done to their "Kama" (fate) when a family member has a handicapping condition. Parents may attribute a birth defect or a handicapping condition to their own behavior during pregnancy and may feel very guilty. Some feel that they need to appeal to God for a "cure." Religious and medical practices common to the Asian minority populations, such as herbal medicine and acupuncture, may be unfamiliar to American professionals. Conversely, many Asian families are unfamiliar with American practices, including speech therapy and rehabilitation, and are reluctant to take their children or family members to clinics or centers for diagnostic or therapeutic services.

Asian language minority adults who need rehabilitative services, such as those who have experienced a cerebrovascular accident or have undergone a laryngectomy, are generally confused and misinformed about the services available to them. Because these patients do not understand the English language, professionals often find it difficult to explain these services to them and to their families. Moreover, professionals are sometimes unaware of certain dynamics in the Asian family or culture and are unprepared to deal with them. For example, although a stroke patient may be better cared for in a convalescent hospital or in a nursing home facility, Asian families may find such a suggestion totally unacceptable because of their culture's emphasis on filial piety.

Recommended Solutions

Speech and hearing professionals need to develop cross-cultural communicative competency, including

- sociocultural knowledge
- linguistic knowledge
- positive attitude toward differences
- flexibility
- communication skills
- mutually congruent interactional competencies

Training programs must be encouraged to take into account the various aspects of bilingualism and multiculturalism and to ensure the following competencies in their graduates:

- the understanding of human communication through the incorporation of resources from psychology, sociology, anthropology, education, linguistics, sociolinguistics, ethnography, special education, multicultural education, and ethnic studies
- the understanding of individual differences through an examination of the issues of integration, assimilation, acculturation, measurement, differences vs. disorders, and acquisition of a second language
- the understanding of cultures and the development of culturally based languages and dialects
- the understanding of sociocultural influences on such communication features as code-switching, turn-taking, voice, fluency, and discourse rules
- the ability to evaluate the language skills of language minority populations by work with interpreters, naturalistic observation, and other methods that do not require a knowledge of the target language
- the ability to adopt, adapt, and create informal test instruments, with the assistance of the speakers of the target language, that are culturally appropriate
- the ability to provide in-service programs to the school, hospitals, and community on the services available to language minority populations
- the knowledge of alternative modes of service to language minority individuals in need of service, such as through a Chinese school, a Japanese school, an Indochinese services center, or a multiservice center
- the ability to collect data and/or conduct research with the intent to improve current practices

The 1985 National Colloquium on Underserved Populations (ASHA, Rockville, Md.) listed the following as areas in need of change to improve service delivery to language minority populations:

1. curriculum development
2. practicum exposure to culturally diverse clients
3. specialty training programs, both professional and paraprofessional
4. paraprofessional training programs for interpreters
5. continuing education to achieve cross-cultural communicative competence
6. flexibility of requirements for cross-cultural communicative competency
7. minority enrollment
8. training of monolingual and/or bilingual minorities to serve multicultural populations
9. recruitment at high school and junior college level
10. encouragement for monolinguals to pursue foreign language proficiency
11. monitoring of foreign language proficiency in those who are bilingual
12. public information to language minority communities
13. research incentives
14. criteria for identifying disorders in language minorities
15. identification of alternative models of service delivery
16. new technological means of service delivery
17. incorporation of specific responsibilities into programs covering language diversity
18. guidelines for determining language proficiency
19. awareness of minority language issues

20. advocacy for clients and families
    - training client advocates
    - increasing education on advocacy for professionals
21. establishment of a Consumer Awareness Board to provide information on tests and materials
22. priority of minority concerns on the national agenda
23. evaluation of federal and state policies

It is unrealistic to expect many current speech-language pathologists and audiologists to acquire linguistic proficiency in one or more of the Asian languages, such as Hmong or Khmer. Adequate speech, language, and hearing services should be provided to Asian language minorities, however. The barriers to the provision of speech, language, and hearing services to the Asian language minority populations are indeed complex. An awareness of the limitations of current services and the need to expand the cultural backgrounds of speech, language, and hearing professionals is the first step toward overcoming these barriers.

CHAPTER 6

Second Language Acquisition

In the 1950s and 1960s, the accepted theoretical explanation of second language learning was based on contrastive analysis. It was asserted that all "errors" made by a second language learner can be explained by reference to the first language (Hyltenstam & Pienemann, 1985). In the late 1960s and early 1970s, however, researchers began to note the limitations of contrastive analysis and concluded that it reveals only one of many possible factors that may affect the learning of a second language.

Corder (1967) postulated that the learning strategies adopted by second language learners are substantially the same as those used to acquire the first language. Researchers in the early 1970s agreed, asserting that second language learners actively construct a grammar for the second language much as they did when they acquired their first language. Emphasis shifted from contrastive analysis toward the larger scope of input theory, in which not only the structure of the mother tongue, but also the structure of any other languages known to the learner and general learning strategies are considered factors in the acquisition of a second language.

Bilingualism

Only 6 of the more than 3,000 languages in the world are spoken by 100 million people, and they are the official languages used by the United Nations: (1) English, (2) French, (3) Russian, (4) Chinese, (5) Arabic, and (6) Spanish. According to the U.S. Bureau of the Census, more than one-tenth of the U.S. population over 4 years of age reports knowing a second language.

The term *bilingual* is derived from the medieval Latin word *lingualis*, which was in turn derived from the Latin word *lingua*, which means tongue. It usually refers to someone who can speak two languages, although it is sometimes used to refer to someone who speaks one language well and understands a second. Koman and Skutnabb-Kangas (1977) delineated three types of bilingualism:

1. proficient bilingualism, or high levels of proficiency in two languages
2. partial bilingualism, or a nativelike level of proficiency in one language and a low level of proficiency in another
3. limited bilingualism, or a low level of proficiency in two languages

Children may acquire proficiency in two languages either simultaneously or sequentially. In simultaneous acquisition, the child is exposed to two languages from birth; in sequential acquisition, the child is exposed to one language from birth and to a second language at a later time. Preschoolers who acquire a second language prior to entering school are considered simultaneous bilinguals. Sequential second language learners range from school-aged children to adults.

Literature on child bilingualism (Boyd, 1974; Ervin-Tripp, 1974; Kessler, 1971; Slobin, 1973) seems to indicate that, regardless of whether the child is a simultaneous or sequential bilingual, the process of acquisition is essentially and structurally similar for the two languages. On the other hand, research seems to indicate that there are some qualitative differences in an adult's acquisition of a second language. For example, sequential second language learners have already acquired a first language and have had a great deal of experience in using that first language in different contexts.

Age Differences in Second Language Acquisition

There are a number of theories regarding the relationship between age and second language learning. Some researchers feel that older second language learners have an advantage over younger ones because the older learners have advanced cognitive development (described by Piaget as the formal operational stage). Most researchers agree that the previous linguistic experience and the cognitive maturity of adult second language learners give them an advantage in terms of the rate of learning. Taylor and Rosansky (cited in Chun, 1980) maintained that factors such as anxiety, motivation, ego boundary, and self-confidence may make adult second language learners more self-conscious, however.

Lenneberg (1967) suggested that there is a critical period after which second language learners are never able to learn and master a second language as they did the first language. Lenneberg felt that postpubescent language learners learn with a "conscious and labored effort" (p. 176). Dulay and Burt (1977) postulated that there is an affective filter in those who are learning a second language. In other words, learners with high anxiety, low motivation, and little self-confidence may have a mental block (affective filter) that prevents them from fully utilizing the input of the language acquisition.

Most researchers agree that the speech of older second language learners is characterized by phonological distortions or a general "foreign accent." Krashen (1981) disagreed with Lenneberg's theory, however. Although he did not see age as a critical factor in the success of second language learning, he felt that children's second language acquisition is effortless and unconscious while adults acquire a second language by conscious learning. Krashen (1981) summarized the age differences in second language acquisition as the following:

1. Older learners are faster in the early stages of second language acquisition because they
   - are better at obtaining comprehensible input (conversational management)
   - have superior knowledge of the world, which helps to make input comprehensible
   - can participate in conversation earlier, via use of first language syntax
2. Younger learners tend to attain higher ultimate levels of proficiency in second languages than do adults because younger learners have a lower affective filter.

Measurement of Language Proficiency

Language minority children typically have much more exposure to English than do their parents. Furthermore, judgments of their proficiency in English are based on a small vocabulary, as well as short and simple sentences, because of their limited repertoire of vocabulary and restricted use of syntax. The proficiency of adult second language learners is judged differently. Adults need to express thoughts unlike those of children, and their speech is more complex and sophisticated. Some common errors of adults may include the misapplication of rules of the second language and oversimplification of morphology and syntax (Ervin-Tripp, 1969).

Language proficiency is commonly measured by certain types of auditory comprehension, speaking, reading comprehension, and writing tasks. Researchers (Bernstein & Tiegerman, 1985; Cheng, 1984; Lund & Duchan, 1983) have argued that measurements of language proficiency should be based on the ability to use language to learn, to communicate, and to meet communicative intent, however. Consequently, they believe that reading or writing tests are not sufficient to measure all the different parameters of communication.

The notion of communicative competence (Hymes, 1971) is defined as the ability to "say the right thing in the right way to the right people in the right place." A set of rules dictates the proper usage of the language and the comprehension of that language. Researchers in speech and language pathology have proposed that assessment of an individual's language ability should include phonology, syntax, morphology, semantics, and pragmatics. Furthermore, Canale (1981, p. 13) has proposed that the following components be assessed:

1. grammatical competence: mastery of appropriate language code
2. sociolinguistic competence: mastery of appropriate language use in different sociolinguistic contexts
3. discourse competence: mastery of ways to combine meanings and forms to achieve a unified text in different modes
4. strategic competence: mastery of verbal and nonverbal strategies (a) to compensate for breakdowns in communication and (b) to enhance communication effectiveness

Factors That Influence Second Language Learning

Both the process and the outcome of second language learning are influenced by several factors:

1. linguistic factors
   - interferences, both phonological (e.g., the substitution of one phoneme for the targeted phoneme) and syntactical (e.g., the use of word order from the first language in the second language)
   - the use of Pidgin English
   - dialect—the need for speakers of other social dialects to become bidialectal
   - comprehensible input

- linguistic intelligence (Gardner, 1983)—ability to learn and use language
- proficiency in the first language
2. sociolinguistic factors
   - amount of exposure to the second language (Wong-Fillmore et al., 1983)
   - speakers of the second language with whom there is contact
   - amount of pressure (peer or familial) to learn the second language
   - age of the learner
3. cultural factors
   - means of survival—the need to use language in making a living
   - perception of the second language
   - need for the second language to ensure academic success
   - isolation from the mainstream
   - identity confusion and cultural conflict
   - country and region of origin
4. psychosocial factors
   - affective filter (Burt & Dulay, 1972)
   - anxiety (Krashen, 1981)
   - motivation
   - self-confidence
   - silent period—a period when second language learners don't say anything
   - adjustment to school or work setting
   - socioeconomic level (Trueba, 1983)
5. educational factors
   - education of the parents
   - views of education
   - educational history (Miramontes, 1984)
6. immigration and family factors
   - time of arrival
   - reason for emigration
   - intervening experiences (e.g., boat, refugee camp)
   - life in other countries
   - life in the country of origin

Although the opinions of researchers regarding second language acquisition differ in many areas, there is some consensus regarding the process. For example, it is generally agreed that first and second language acquisitions involve essentially universal cognitive strategies. Moreover, errors of various types are better described in terms of these learning strategies than in terms of interferences, even though some errors can be attributed to interferences. A single linguistic system forms the basis for language acquisition, storage, and retrieval of both first and second languages. Children need to have input that is meaningful to them; the quality and quantity of comprehensible input determine the success of second language acquisition. Finally, it is agreed that, because learning a second language is a (gradual) process, it may take 4 to 7 years for learners to become proficient in the second language.

English as a Foreign Language in the United States

Cummins (1981), Krashen et al. (1979), Wong-Fillmore (1984), and Genesee (1978) maintained that the following factors influence the outcome of the language minority students' effort to learn English:

1. prestige of the native language
2. security of the children's identity and self-concept
3. level of support for the development of the first language at home
4. language spoken at home
5. level of support for the development of the first language in the environment (e.g., school, community)
6. age on arrival in the United States

Categories of Second Language Learners

There are several different categories of second language learners in the United States:

1. adult immigrants and refugees (i.e., sequential second language learners), including
   - immigrants who have come to the United States for education or employment and have received instruction in English prior to their arrival
   - immigrants who have come to the United States to join family members (e.g., spouse, parents), and may not have had previous training in English
   - refugees who were forced to leave their home countries because of political, economic, or other difficulties, the majority of whom do not know any English
   - illegal aliens who have come to the United States to seek a better living, the majority of whom do not know any English
2. foreign-born children (ranging from infants to adolescents) who are unfamiliar with the English language, including
   - children whose parents came to the United States for further study and employment
   - children who have come to the United States as refugees either through the arrangement of an American sponsor or an agency
   - children who have come to the United States as refugees through the sponsorship of a parent or a relative
3. second generation American-born children, including
   - children whose parents are well-educated, permanent residents of the United States and use English in the home
   - children whose parents are unable to speak much English and use the mother tongue and Pidgin English at home
   - children whose parents came to the United States as refugees, are unable to speak any English, and use the mother tongue at home.
4. third generation American-born children, including
   - children whose parents speak both English and the mother tongue and code-switch (i.e., simultaneous second language learners)
   - children whose parents speak only English

- children who are cared for by their grandparents who speak the mother tongue and by their parents who speak English or code-switch (i.e., simultaneous second language learners)

Because of the variety of environments in which these groups learn, it is difficult to make general statements about their language learning processes. All want to communicate effectively and to achieve nativelike communicative competence, however. Wong-Fillmore (1985) pointed out that "there is quite certainly some rock-bottom level of exposure required to sustain a language learning effort at all, . . . and there is most certainly a minimum level of social contact with English speakers that is required to achieve this" (p. 439).

In assessing the language dominance and the language proficiency of the second language learner in the United States, it is critical to ask the following questions:

1. How old was the individual when he or she came to the United States?
2. Has the individual had training in English before entering the United States? If yes:
   - How many years of training?
   - Where was the training?
   - Who was the trainer?
   - How was the training done?
3. If the individual is a child immigrant or refugee:
   - Do his or her parents speak English at home?
   - Does he or she speak a language other than English at home? If yes, to whom? what language(s)?
   - Do his or her siblings speak English at home? If not, what languages do they speak at home?
   - Does he or she speak English with playmates? If not, what languages do they use to communicate?
4. If the individual is an adult refugee:
   - What language is used at home?
   - Is English required in the work setting (e.g., factory, restaurant)?
   - If the individual does not understand English, who talks for the individual when English is needed (e.g., at meetings with school personnel)?
   - If the individual does not read English, who translates for him or her?
   - How often is English required in his or her daily living?
   - In terms of social activities, how often is English used?
5. If the individual is a second generation American-born child:
   - What is the language(s) used at home?
   - What language(s) do the parents use to speak to each other?
   - Do the parents speak English to the child?
   - Do the grandparents speak English to the child?

Instruction in English as a Second Language

In the environment of an American elementary or secondary school, Asian language minority students of limited English proficiency (LEP) learn English as a second language (ESL) through (1) formal instruction and (2) informal practice outside the language class. Because many parents of the Asian language minority students do not speak English at all or do not speak English well, the students must use their native language to communicate at home and in their community. This lack of practice in English at home makes it necessary for them to have a great deal of formal instruction and informal practice at school before they can develop communicative competence in English.

Language minority students learn to use English to communicate with their teachers, classmates, and friends, both inside and outside their classroom. They learn to use the English language in a natural and experiential way. In the education of these students, both ESL teachers and classroom teachers are key figures. They not only impart factual knowledge, but also provide modeling and training for the use of language to synthesize and create meaningful ideas. There are conflicts caused by the students' lack of awareness of the differences between the rules at home and at school, and the incorporation of new behaviors and the associated values is a significant struggle for the students. Teachers who observe the overt behaviors that reflect this struggle often misinterpret them as signs of disinterest. Instead, however, teachers should serve as bridge builders in nurturing the development of appropriate new behaviors and minimizing such conflicts.

The ESL class provides students with drills on the basic structures and articulation of the English language. Furthermore, ESL materials are designed to introduce vocabulary idioms and prosodic (segmental and suprasegmental) features to the students. Important aspects of American culture and the pragmatic use of the language are also part of the ESL curriculum. When ESL classes are not available to the language minority students, special arrangements are generally made for tutoring.

Wong-Fillmore (1983) noted two major functions of the language used by teachers of LEP students: (1) to impart to their students the information and skills that the students are supposed to be learning in school and (2) to provide the linguistic input on which these students can base their language learning. According to Wong-Fillmore (1983), effective teaching of LEP students requires

1. clear separation of languages (i.e., no alternation or mixing)
2. an emphasis on comprehension and a focus on communication through demonstration, enactment to convey meaning, the presentation of new information in the context of known information, and message redundancy
3. grammatical use of language appropriate to an activity, including the use of similar structures, avoidance of complex structures, repeated use of the same sentence patterns or routines, and the use of paraphrase for variation
4. tailoring of elicitation questions to allow for different levels of participation from students
5. demonstration of the richness of language by use of material not in books and playfulness

In summary, Wong-Fillmore indicated that teachers should focus on helping students to develop a greater command of the forms, functions, and uses of the English language.

There are different types of second language learners (Wong-Fillmore, 1985). Some are super learners, and some take time in learning. For all types of learners, Wong-Fillmore noted, the extent of exposure to the English language is critical to the pace of language learning. Kiraithe (1985) maintained that words must be heard more than 200 times before they finally become part of a learner's repertoire. She also indicated that those learning a second language go through a period of "silence" during which they just absorb the language by listening.

Researchers, such as Cummins (1981), have reported that language minority students take much longer to approach commonly accepted age/grade norms in context-reduced aspects of English proficiency (4 to 7 years on the average) than in context-embedded aspects (2 years on the average). In other words, students learn from contextual cues, and the reduction of such cues reduces comprehension (Figure 6-1). Cummins (1981) maintained that everyday communication is informal and context-embedded, whereas classroom interactions are more formal and context-reduced (Figure 6-2). Thus, language minority children may appear to be English-proficient in casual conversation, but fail in mainstream classrooms where context-reduced communication strategies are expected and rewarded.

According to Cummins (1981), the communicative demands of schooling and the acquisition of literacy and academic skills require more than daily face-to-face, one-to-one communication. The American way of schooling requires such strategies as responding in terms of the logic of the text rather than in terms of prior knowledge, asking questions, and volunteering comments—all strategies that are learned, context-bound, and culture-specific. It is necessary to examine the English proficiency of Asian language minority students from both the perspective of basic interpersonal and communicative skills and cognitive academic linguistic skills (Cummins, 1978). Research in the areas of pragmatics and ethnography (Bedrosian, 1985; Iglesias, 1985; Lund & Duchan, 1983; Prutting, 1982; Ripich & Spinelli, 1985) has confirmed the need to include multiple levels, multi-

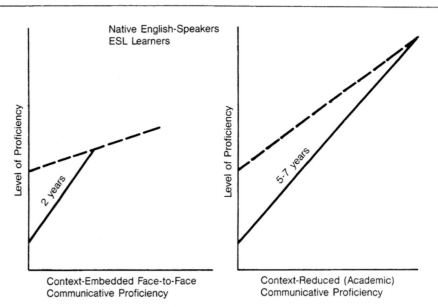

Figure 6-1 Length of Time Required to Achieve Age-Appropriate Levels of Context-Embedded and Context-Reduced Communicative Proficiency

Source: From *Schooling and Language Minority Students: A Theoretical Framework* (p. 16) by California State Department of Education, Office of Bilingual Bicultural Education (Ed.), 1981, Los Angeles, Ca.: California State University, Evaluation, Dissemination and Assessment Center. Reprinted by permission.

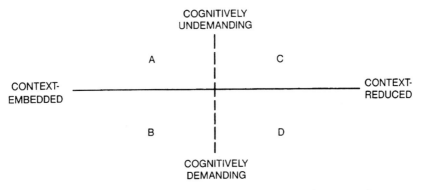

Figure 6-2 Range of Contextual Support and Degree of Cognitive Involvement in Communicative Activities

Source: From *Schooling and Language Minority Students: A Theoretical Framework* by California State Department of Education, Office of Bilingual Bicultural Education (Ed.), 1981, Los Angeles, Ca.: California State University, Evaluation, Dissemination and Assessment Center. Reprinted by permission.

---

ple partners, and multiple contexts in the evaluation of the language ability of an individual.

Development of Cross-Cultural Communicative Competence
Speech, language, and hearing professionals need to develop their cross-cultural communicative competence in order to meet the needs of their culturally diverse clients. The concept of cross-cultural communicative competence has five important elements:

1. communication skills, including sensitivity and awareness of interactive styles
2. sociocultural knowledge (i.e., knowledge of the values and beliefs of other cultures, including their concept of kinship, family patterns, and appropriate social proximity)
3. linguistic knowledge (i.e., basic knowledge of the five linguistic domains of the client's native language—phonology, morphology, syntax, semantics, and pragmatics), including paralinguistic knowledge (e.g., nonverbal communication, kinesics, and proxemics) and metalinguistic knowledge (i.e., the use of language to comment about language)
4. sense of cultural relativism (i.e., recognition that all languages and cultures are qualitatively equal) and an appreciation of the commonalities, as well as the differences, among peoples, cultures, and languages
5. mutually congruent interactional competence (i.e., the ability to recognize a need for elaboration and clarification and to provide such when meaning is unclear)

According to Hunsaker and Alessandra (1980), there are four main interactive styles in communication: (1) amiable, (2) expressive, (3) analytical, and (4) driving. Schematically, these interactive styles can be represented by four quadrants, each of which contains characteristic traits (Exhibit 6-1).The amiable type talks slowly, responds slowly, is more reserved, and tends to agree with what others say. The expressive type generally talks and responds quickly, and is

Exhibit 6-1 Predominant Characteristics of Each Behavioral Style

High Responsiveness

Amiable Style	*Expressive Style*
Slow at taking action and making decisions	Spontaneous actions and decisions
Likes close, personal relationships	Likes involvement
Dislikes interpersonal conflict	Dislikes being alone
Supports and "actively" listens to others	Exaggerates and generalizes
Weak at goal setting and self-direction	Tends to dream and get others caught up in his dream
Has excellent ability to gain support from others	Jumps from one activity to another
Works slowly and cohesively with others	Works quickly and excitedly with others
Seeks security and belongingness	Seeks esteem and belongingness
Good counseling skills	Good persuasive skills

Low Assertiveness———————————————————————**High Assertiveness**

Analytical Style	*Driver Style*
Cautious actions and decisions	Firm actions and decisions
Likes organization and structure	Likes control
Dislikes involvement with others	Dislikes inaction
Asks many questions about specific details	Prefers maximum freedom to manage himself and others
Prefers objective, task-oriented, intellectual work environment	Cool and independent; competition with others
Wants to be right and therefore relies too much on data collection	Low tolerance for feelings, attitudes, and advice of others
Works slowly and precisely alone	Works quickly and impressively by himself
Seeks security and self-actualization	Seeks esteem and self-actualization
Good problem-solving skills	Good administrative skills

Low Responsiveness

Source: From *The Art of Managing People* (p. 35–36) by P.L. Hunsaker and A.J. Alessandra, 1980, New York: Simon & Schuster, Inc. Copyright © 1980 by P.L. Hunsaker and A.J. Alessandra. Reprinted by permission of Simon & Schuster, Inc.

highly verbal and spontaneous. The analytical type generally appears to be reserved and calculating, and is more precise and detail-oriented. The driver type is less verbal and more action-oriented, and tends to be direct and straightforward in manner.

A sensitivity to clients' cultural background, together with an awareness of the various interactive styles, will enhance the practitioner's understanding of the reasons behind some of the clients' overt and observed behaviors. For example, the Asian cultural emphasis on respect for the elderly and teachers affects the behavior of Asian language minority children in school. Asian children are expected to be amiable in their interactive style, doing as they are told, without argument. As a result, individuals working with Asian children must be patient and help them to say what they really want to say rather than what they think the teacher wants to hear. It is also important for teachers to determine what these children want to do, since they will generally follow commands and directions without argument. The idea of following their personal inclinations never occurs to some of them. Even when they feel a strong aversion to a particular task, their desire for teacher approval is even stronger. Thus, educators may need to probe and provide an opportunity for Asian students to choose a desired task.

Educators' knowledge of another culture is incomplete until they know the organization of the family system and the function of the kinship system. In order to communicate effectively with family members it is necessary to know who makes the decisions in the family. It is also necessary to understand the family hierarchy and the child-rearing practices of that culture. Furthermore, educators must be sensitive to the possible conflicts on child-rearing between the child's parents or between the child's grandparents and the child's parents. Such intergenerational conflicts of cultural practice may lead to communication breakdowns between the first generation immigrants (grandparents) and their children (parents) and failure of compliance with the older generations' expectations.

Writings of LEP Students

Some language minority LEP students find it difficult to express themselves as they cope with the conflicting values from home and school; feel isolated and alienated, disappointed and embarrassed; sense prejudices and rejections; and feel confused and lost. Others are able to highlight their difficulties and feelings clearly, as shown in these excerpts from *Refugee Update*:

. . . Now, that I'm here, I noticed that it wasn't all true. I wish people would understand that we are here because of the war. We were in the war helping the Americans and their allies. I wish people would try to understand; instead, of being prejudiced. I now understand that not all Americans accept me into the United States. Americans and everyone should try to understand us refugees. If I can have a good education and get a good job, I would rather work than live on Welfare all my life. I can make my future here, too. War could not beat me and neither will prejudice. (Cha Vang, 10th grade, Hmong, in U.S. 5 years)

. . . I hear the popcorns are calling my name, and we are almost through. Then my nose starts to smell oil and butter all over the place. It looks crunchy and hot. My mouth starts to swallow my tongue through my throat, and my stomach starts to scream. It will taste delicious. I feel like I already swallow my teeth through my throat. I ask my mom to put the popcorn quickly in the bowl for me. Finally, she puts it in the bowl. She gives the bowl to me; I take it to the living room, and find a comfortable place to sit on . . . (May Vang, 12th grade, Hmong, in U.S. 5 years)

My first day in an American school was one of the worst days in my life. I was already familiar to the machines, automobiles, people, but not the school. It was completely different from my country. I had Physical Education for first period. The teacher did not care if you understand or not any English. She just kept talking and asking me a lot of questions. I was very afraid to ask any questions about what we were doing. Therefore, the only way out was to follow the American students, and do what they were doing. I thought I was going to have all classes with American students, where the teacher did not care about the people that don't know, where all the kids laugh and tease you about what you say or do. I was very surprised with my second period class. They did not stare at me like I was a different human being. I was surrounded by Asian students, and I heard different languages in that classroom. The teacher had always a big smile on her face that showed compassion and patience; she made sure that we understood every sentence that she said. She made me feel relieved and comfortable in that class. All the students were helping each other and working together as a family. We were all in the same level; therefore, no one could tease me about my mistakes. (Carla Chang, 9th grade; Taiwanese, Spanish, Portuguese; in the U.S. 1½ years)*

The following letters from a book entitled *Dear Diane: Letters from Our Daughters* (Yen-Mei Wong, 1983) provide additional perspective on the feelings of some of these youngsters:

Dear Diane: My parents embarrass me to no end. We were coming home from a visit to relatives and stopped at a roadside restaurant to eat. They attracted so much attention, I just could've died. They spoke Chinese loudly the whole time and slurped their soup, just like they were at home. I'm so glad none of my friends were there; it was bad enough having all those strangers staring at us. Do you have any suggestions on how to get them to behave like normal people?

Dear Diane: I'm an American-born Korean student. Some white students think I'm a foreigner, even though I speak only English and wear normal clothes. If I hang around with my mom's Korean friends and families, I'll be worse off than I am already. What can I do?

Dear Diane: At school, teachers tell us to ask questions and to challenge what they say. At home, it's just the opposite. Whenever I offer an opinion that is different than what my folks think, they say I'm rude and disobedient. I suppose that I can remain silent in front of them, but isn't there a way that I can express my opinions without them raising the roof?

Dear Diane: My parents always tell me they want me to be a doctor, lawyer, or engineer. They say that the only reason they came to America was so that I could go to a good school and then get a good job. I can't handle the pressure and feel guilty because I can't live up to their expectations. I resent them because they don't seem to appreciate what I've done. I don't want to live their lives.

Dear Diane: Just before the end of the school year, my mom gave me a small gift to take to my teacher. It was only a box of stationery with some Korean designs. I was so upset. My teacher refused to accept the gift and told me that she was not taking any "bribes" from any Koreans, or anyone else. I didn't know what to say. What's wrong with me? What can I do about the teacher?*

Difficulties vs. Disorders

More research is needed on the acquisition of a second language. Speech, language, and hearing professionals need to broaden their knowledge base about the normal process of second language learning in order to differentiate normal difficulties in language learning from language disorders.

Normal Difficulties of Language Learners

Second language learners encounter numerous difficulties in the learning process. These difficulties are normal and should not be viewed as aberrant. Each individual has a unique experience in language learning and a unique perception of his or her own abilities. From the reports, writings, and interviews

---

*From *Refugee Update*, January 1986.

of second language learners, practitioners can get a general impression of the normal second language learning process.

Some Asian LEP students speak their first language at home and in their neighborhood, hearing English only in school. Some speak their first language at school with children who came from the same country. Others hear English more often, as they have neighbors and friends who speak English.

Language Learning Disorders

Case #1

A Laotian child, aged 2 years and 7 months, was referred for an initial speech and language evaluation because he formed no intelligible words. The pregnancy history appeared normal. The child's bilirubin level had been high enough to require a 3-day hospitalization immediately after birth, however, and he had a history of a mild ear infection in his first year. He achieved his gross motor milestones within normal limits. His parents described him as a quiet child who enjoyed watching television. In general, he did not seem to enjoy toys, although he liked to play with blocks.

The child lived with his parents and three older siblings. Laotian was the language spoken at home, although the three older children generally spoke English among themselves and spoke Laotian to their parents. The parents reported that the child seemed uninterested in talking and did not seem to enjoy the company of other children. Very worried and frustrated about the child's lack of language, the parents were concerned that the child's problems in learning Laotian originated in confusion about the use of two languages, English and Laotian, in the home. They believed that they might have to use English in order to provide a more consistent way of communication.

Observation. In the testing room, the child was quiet. Although several toys had been arranged around the room, he showed no interest in them. The child went to the desk, picked up a cup of water that had been placed on the desk, and took it to his seat. He found another cup in a kitchen toy and started to pour the water from one cup to the other; he continued to pour the water back and forth, seeming to enjoy the activity. When asked to look at some pictures, the child did not respond. When asked to play with a doll, the child simply turned away.

When the clinician took away the cups, the child threw a temper tantrum. He pulled his hair and even bit himself during the temper tantrum. His behavior seemed difficult to control. His parents commented that he cried and threw temper tantrums from time to time. The only way that they could calm him down was to take him for a ride, the motion of the car put him to sleep.

Attempts at formal testing were unsuccessful, as the child responded very little to the various stimuli presented. Because he enjoyed playing with blocks, the parents were asked to bring the blocks from home to the clinic. The child played with the blocks by arranging them in different orders. Occasionally, he happened to spell a word with the blocks.

When the child noticed a jar of tongue depressors in the corner of the room, he went to the jar, opened it, and took out a tongue depressor. Giving the depressor to the clinician, he quickly opened his mouth. The clinician was able to do a through oral peripheral examination. The results of the examination were within normal limits. Observing this, the mother remarked that the child had frequent ear, nose, and throat examinations at the doctor's office, and he seemed to know the routine. In fact, he actually insisted on such an examination each time he visited the doctor.

Over an observation period of 3 months, the child made no vocalization, except for an occasional outburst of crying. Attempts to elicit vocalization were unsuccessful. The mother later reported that she heard the child saying ''dog'' at home; when the clinician attempted to elicit the word from the child, however, she was unsuccessful.

Clinical Impressions. The fact that the three components of language (i.e., form, function, content) were equally depressed made it clear that the child's problem in communication went beyond the lack of language exposure, as the parents suspected. The lack of language form (i.e., phonology, morphology, and syntax) certainly was a concern to the clinician, as well as to the parents. Communicative intent and language comprehension, the semantic domain of language, also seemed to be lacking, however. The clinician diagnosed the child's communication problem as autism, based on the following observations over a period of time:

1. a pragmatic deficit in that the child failed to initiate or maintain any type of communication with his parents, his siblings, or the clinician. The child showed no behavior that would indicate any intent to communicate.
2. a lack of semantic development in that the child did not seem to comprehend language, since the child did not generally follow commands or instructions. Expression was absent.
3. an apparent delay in phonological development. Since the child said nothing during the sessions, the clinician could not assess phonological development; however, the lack of output suggested a delay in phonology.
4. a delay in syntactical and morphological development in that the child said nothing.
5. the following behavioral characteristics:
   - gaze aversion. The child had no eye contact with other people during interaction.
   - ritualistic behavior. The child seemed to manipulate objects in his environment in a ritualistic fashion, such as pouring water in and out of cups.
   - temper tantrums. The child's temper tantrums were self-abusive, and the onset of such tantrums was generally sudden.
   - self-stimulatory behavior. The child seemed to enjoy sucking his thumb and looking at the ceiling for long, long periods of time.
   - hyposensitivity to stimuli. The mother reported that the child did not seem to feel pain and even had a high tolerance for hot food, being able to eat a whole jar of hot peppers without any difficulty.
   - reciprocity. The child seemed not to use communicative exchange at all. He produced no sounds or words during the clinical observation, although the mother reported that he said a few words at home. Those were very unexpected, however, and he never seemed to say the same words again.

Outcome. The parent conference was held after several observation sessions. A speech-language clinician, a psychologist, and a pediatrician who specialized in behavioral problems together informed the parents of the diagnosis of autism. The parents appeared passive and unresponsive, and it was difficult for the clinicians to elicit responses or comments from them. When asked whether they understood what the clinicians were saying, the parents generally nodded their heads and answered, "Yes, yes." The clinicians asked whether the parents were frustrated and angry, but the parents denied that they were.

The cultural aspect of the conference required a great deal of attention. The cultural barriers to communication, as well as the parents' attitudes in spousal communication, made it difficult to convey all the messages successfully. The clinicians and counselors were hoping for a two-way communication, while the Oriental parents expected a one-way communication from authorities. When the clinician wanted to work *with* the parents in examining alternate strategies, the parents were uncomfortable as participants in the decision-making process. Their understanding of autism was far from complete, and they were actually disappointed when the clinician did not simply recommend a course of action without seeking their opinion. The clinician's loosely defined patterns of interaction also irritated the parents somewhat. As Asians, they expected a clear and well-defined pattern of interaction between clinician and client.

The parents had difficulty conducting an open discussion about their feelings. The clinicians were familiar with autistic behaviors; however, the parents were a little confused, thinking that the child looked physically normal, and could not seem to understand that a normal-looking child could have a neurological problem. Their passive appearance and their seemingly uninvolved attitude made it very difficult for the clinicians to work with them constructively and successfully.

Because the clinician understood the communication styles and the cultures of the parents, the cultural barriers slowly gave way. The child was later placed in a public school, where the teachers also worked very closely with the parents. Over several months the parents began to communicate more with the school authorities and the medical specialists.

Case #2

A Vietnamese child was referred for a speech and language evaluation when he was 2 years and 6 months old because he was slow in acquiring language. Birth history and pregnancy appeared normal, and the child's medical history and developmental history seemed uneventful. He was one of three children. According to the mother, his 7-year-old brother occasionally stuttered, and his older sister had talked very late. The child did not start talking until he was 2 years and 3 months old.

The child's parents worked; the mother had two jobs and was seldom at home. The grandmother, who spoke Vietnamese to him, cared for the child while the parents worked. Vietnamese was the language spoken at home.

According to the mother, the child was a good eater and played well with other children. In his immediate environment, he had his brother to play with. During the day, his cousins played with him, and they all spoke Vietnamese. The mother further indicated that the child sometimes watched the other children play and seemed to have difficulty understanding their activities. At the time of the examination, he was saying a few single words intelligibly, such as mama and papa.

Observation. The clinician could not speak or understand Vietnamese; she asked the mother to play with the child and simply observed their interactions. Because the mother appeared to be uneasy playing with the child, the clinician asked the mother if she played with the child at home. The mother said that she was too busy working two jobs. As the grandmother was present at the session, she was asked to play with the child. She simply responded to the mother, "I don't play with the child. He plays by himself." Both the mother and the grandmother seemed rather quiet and reserved.

The child's brother was in the clinic, and the clinician asked the brother to play with the child. The brother seemed quite good at telling the child what he was doing. The child mimicked his brother and occasionally repeated a word that his brother had said.

The clinician asked the mother to bring the child's cousin, who was the same age, to a session. The child's cousin was immediately fascinated by the bowling set. Using very simple English, the clinician explained to the children how to place the pins and how to throw the bowling ball to hit the pins. Both children seemed to understand that they had to take turns lining up the pins and throwing the ball. Although they did not understand the rules behind the bowling game, they seemed very interested in throwing the ball and hitting the pins.

The child's cousin imitated and repeated some of the words the clinician said in English. Although both were very involved in the bowling activity, the children exchanged very little conversation. The cousin did talk to his aunt, the child's mother, in Vietnamese about how he liked the game. He used short sentences of two or three words. Comparing the child's speech and his cousin's speech, the clinician noticed a wide gap in the length of their utterances.

Clinical Impressions. Because of the child's youth at the time of testing, the clinician chose to use informal observation to assess the child's language development. The child seemed to have difficulty labeling objects, both in Vietnamese and in English. He did imitate many words that the clinician uttered, however. Although his attempts to imitate polysyllabic words were unsuccessful, his repetition of simple words was generally quite adequate. In terms of auditory comprehension, the child was having some difficulty following two-level commands (for example, go to the door and pick up the book), but was able to follow one-level commands (for example, give me the block). When the child wanted something, he usually used gestures. His overall utterances were very restricted and limited.

Examination of oral-speech mechanism revealed structures to be within normal limits. The child seemed alert and appeared to be cooperative. His attention span was short; he jumped from one activity to another.

Outcome. It was concluded that the child exhibited a language problem in his native language. The clinician felt that the child probably did not have many opportunities to interact socially with multiple partners and that language stimulation at home would be a most essential part of the remediation program. The clinician spent a great deal of time with the mother and the grandmother, explaining child language development. Although the grandmother did not understand English, the mother was able to translate the explanations for the child's grandmother. Given the right linguistic and social environment, it was felt that the child would improve.

During the observation period, it became clear that the child's inability to speak hindered his relationship with the father in that the father almost refused to take the child anywhere. After 9 months of the home program and therapy (which was done in English), the father felt more comfortable with the child. The ability to communicate effectively seemed to be a crucial factor in strengthening the bond between father and son. As a consequence, the child began to talk about the father during sessions, whereas in the past he had almost always referred only to the mother and the grandmother. Furthermore, increased interaction with the father helped improve the overall communication at home.

The child's inability to produce output at one point in time was not sufficient evidence for a diagnosis of a language disorder. The child had a comprehensible input in the environment and exposure for language development. Once the parents and the grandmother began to involve the child actively in social interaction, the child was able to learn Vietnamese quite readily. The child's acquisition of English was slower because his exposure was less frequent. His development of English seemed within the normal range, however.

The clinician's understanding of the home background, as well as the home culture, of the child, helped to make the parent-clinician relationship more comfortable. In this case, the parents were educated and could speak and understand English well, and the clinician attempted to learn a few words in Vietnamese so that she could communicate with the grandmother. The home program provided by the clinician seemed effective. The child's growth in language encouraged the mother and father to continue providing adequate language stimulation at home.

The clinician became more of a consultant than a therapist in this case, although she did spend some time working with the child in the clinic. Even though her ability to understand the language of the child was very limited, she was effective in providing professional information to the parents, thus contributing to the success of the program.

PART III

Evaluation of the Skills of Language Minority Speakers

CHAPTER 7

A Team Approach to Assessment

The 1985–1986 update survey of the American Speech-Language-Hearing Association (ASHA) indicates that there are no certified speech-language pathologists and audiologists in the United Sates who speak Vietnamese, Laotian, Khmer, Tagalog, Hmong, Korean, or Yiu-Mienh. There are only a few bilingual speech-language pathologists and audiologists who speak some of the other, more widely used Asian languages, such as Chinese and Japanese. As a result, the speech and language problems of Asian children are sometimes not identified. Many of these children are mislabeled as learning-disabled and placed in special education classes. Among the professionals who are members of the special education team, however, few comprehend or speak any of the Asian languages.

Because the federal mandate requires that the abilities of children with limited English proficiency (LEP) be assessed in their native language, speech-language pathologists and audiologists need to develop their competencies in the assessment of these students. The California Commission for Teacher Preparation and Licensing (*California Speech and Hearing Association Newsletter*, 1985) recommended the following competencies for bilingual speech-language specialists:

I. *Second Language Competencies*
   Language competency will be satisfied by completion of a language proficiency test with 80% accuracy in both oral and written language skills. The skills include:
   A. The ability to understand and engage in informational conversation.
   B. The ability to read an average length paragraph and answer questions.
   C. The ability to write an average length paragraph using correct grammatical structures.

II. *Competencies in Relation to Cultural Variables*
   Speech-language specialists should develop an awareness of the existence of cultural similarities and differences to include:
   A. Family structure (relation of child to parents/siblings).
   B. Community (relation of child to own community).
   C. Urban acculturation (urbanization-community participation).

    D. Nonacademic roles (what is expected of child at home, etc., in nonacademic situations).

    E. Self-maintenance (caring for oneself).

In order to achieve these objectives, the California Commission suggested a team approach that uses resources from related professions (e.g., sociology, anthropology, linguistics).

  III. *Competencies in the Area of Language Development*
    A. Knowledge of universal language milestones.
    B. Knowledge of language acquisition in primary language.
    C. Knowledge of the continua for second language acquisition, to include contrastive analysis of phonemic and syntactic systems.
    D. Knowledge of the cognitive and language development of a normally-developing bilingual child.
    E. Knowledge of cultural factors, to include semantic and pragmatic systems as they relate to sociolinguistic environment [e.g., parent-child, school-child interaction].

  IV. *Competencies in the Area of Assessment*
    A. Ability to complete interviews with parents of children of different cultural backgrounds. [Refer to Competencies in Section II.]
    B. Ability to verify the language dominance of a pupil.
    C. Ability to determine the language proficiency of a pupil through observation, test administration.
    D. Ability to evaluate and interpret existing test instruments.
    E. Ability to devise or adapt existing instruments for assessing LES/NES [limited English-speaking/non-English-speaking] pupils.
      a. develop new normative data appropriate to the population.
      b. develop criterion-referenced instrument appropriate to the population.

  V. *Responsibilities of Speech-Language Specialists to Translator*
    A. Must achieve proficiencies as defined in Section I of Second Language Competencies.

Additional competencies should include:
    B. Understanding of child development.
    C. Understanding of speech and language development and positive attributes of bilingualism.
    D. Knowledge of testing procedures, test instruments, test behaviors.
    E. Understanding of cross-cultural variables.
    F. Understanding of the role and responsibilities of the translator.

The California Commission has suggested using these definitions:

Language proficiency. Near native fluency in both the minority language and the English language.

Normative processes. Ability to describe the process of normal speech and language acquisition for both bilingual and monolingual individuals; and how those processes are manifested in oral and written language.

Assessment. Ability to administer and interpret formal and informal assessment procedures to distinguish between communication differences and communication disorders.

Intervention. Ability to apply intervention strategies for treatment of communicative disorders in the minority language.

Cultural sensitivity. Ability to recognize cultural factors that affect the delivery of speech-language pathology and audiology services to the minority language-speaking community.

As noted previously, it is unrealistic to expect that there will be in the near future a sufficient number of trained bilingual speech-language professionals to serve the Asian language minority population. Therefore, it may be necessary to conduct assessments and provide services through a team approach, including the use of interpreters and/or translators.

Role of the Interpreter/Translator

Ideally, bilingual/bicultural speech, language, and hearing professionals provide services in the primary language of their clients. Because of the extreme shortage of bilingual/bicultural professionals trained to serve Asian language minority populations, monolingual professionals must take the responsibility of selecting and training interpreters and translators.

The ASHA recommends the use of interpreters or translators to collect assessment data on the language skills of language minority speakers if the certified speech-language pathologist or audiologist on the staff does not meet the recommended competencies to provide services to speakers of limited English proficiency (LEP), if an individual who needs services speaks a language that is uncommon for that local area, or if there are no trained professionals readily available with proficiency in that language that would permit the use of other strategies. Individuals who could serve as interpreters or translators include (1) professional interpreters or translators from language banks or services, (2) bilingual professional staff from a health or education discipline other than communicative disorders, (3) a member of the client's community who has been trained as an interpreter or translator, or, when there is no trained interpreter or translator available, (4) a family member or friend of the client, or (5) a student from the same school who is proficient in the home language of the student.

Interpretation vs. Translation

It is important to differentiate between an interpreter and a translator, although most people use the two terms interchangeably. Interpretation refers to oral communication; the spoken message is converted from one language to another language. Translation refers to written communication; the written message is converted from one language to another language. The role of an interpreter/translator (I/T) goes beyond the word-for-word conversion of messages, however; it includes explanation and clarification. In interacting with Asian language minority populations, interpretation/translation is often needed.

In general, there are three types of *interpretation:*

1. consecutive interpretation. The interpreter listens to the message in language 1 (L1) pauses for a moment, and converts the message into language 2 (L2). Speakers should not talk in long, complicated sentences, but rather in short and meaningful units. Testing and parent conferences are conducted primarily by consecutive interpretation.

2. simultaneous interpretation. The interpreter provides an immediate interpretation of what is being said. The interpreter must be able to recall long units and instantly supply a synonym for any specific word that he or she does not know. This type of interpretation is very difficult and requires extensive training. Highly skilled professionals at the United Nations do this kind of interpretation.

3. whispered interpretation. The interpreter sits next to the person for whom he or she is interpreting in a meeting or conference and whispers interpretations to the person as the meeting proceeds.

There are two types of *translation:*

1. prepared translation. The translator has time before the actual contact to read the materials and to obtain clarification or check with the dictionary so that he or she is prepared for the translation.

2. sight translation. The translator is given written material and asked to translate it on the spot.

Prerequisites for Interpretation/Translation

Not everyone who speaks two languages can be an I/T. Proficiency in two languages is indeed a prerequisite, but it is not sufficient for someone to function successfully as an I/T. In addition to the ability to convert from L1 to L2 and vice versa, the I/T needs a good memory in order to retain information and the ability to supply other words with the same meaning when the specific words cannot be retrieved. For this, the I/T needs some knowledge about the terminology of the topic at hand, such as speech and language disorders, hearing impairment, or cerebral palsy. The I/T should be willing to ask for clarification or repetition of the message if he or she is unclear about the meaning, however. The I/T may also need to take notes of key points made during the entire process so that these points can be highlighted appropriately.

The I/T needs to have a good rapport with people and a knowledge of the rules of social interaction in the two cultures. A pragmatic knowledge of the two cultures helps the I/T to understand (1) that the same words sometimes have different meanings in the two languages; (2) that words in one language cannot always be translated into another language because there is no parallel concept; and (3) that nonverbal, vocal, tonal, and intonational cues, as well as gestures, facial expressions, and body language must be taken into consideration. The I/T must be conscious of this paralinguistic information. Furthermore, the I/T should be trained to adjust to the different levels of language use (e.g., conversational, formal, informal, colloquial, idiomatic).

The I/T must remain neutral. He or she should not editorialize, change, or make corrections, but should be faithful to what the speaker says or writes. Although there may be occasions on which the I/T disagrees with the speaker, the I/T must remember that he or she is there not to make a judgment, but to interpret.

An interpretation is only as good as the original. I/Ts typically make the following types of mistakes:

1. omissions. I/Ts may omit single words, phrases, or sentences, generally when
   • they do not know the meaning of the words, phrases, or sentences

- the words cannot be translated
- they cannot keep up with the pace of the speaker
- they cannot retain all the details and have forgotten what was said
- the words appear to be of no importance (e.g., very, rather)

2. additions. I/Ts may add extra words, phrases, or entire sentences, generally when
   - they wish to be more elaborate
   - they editorialize
   - they need to explain a difficult concept for which there is no equivalent in the other language

3. substitutions. I/Ts may use words, phrases, or sentences other than the specified ones, generally when
   - they make an error
   - they misunderstand the speaker
   - they cannot keep up with the pace of the speaker and must make up material based on the words that they have heard
   - they are confused about the words (e.g., homonyms)
   - they fail to retrieve a specific word or phrase;
   - they use an incorrect reference.

4. transformations. I/Ts may change the word order of the statement, sometimes distorting the meanings.

5. errors resulting from unequal skills in L1 or L2. I/Ts may find it easier to interpret from L1 to L2 than from L2 to L1.

6. errors resulting from idiosyncratic style. I/Ts may change the meaning of the message through their idiosyncrasy in intonation, facial expressions, and gestures.

The I/T should understand the need for confidentiality. Ideally, the I/T should be familiar with the confidentiality procedures and policies of the school, agency, or setting in which the interpretation or translation is taking place. In order to maintain professionalism, the I/T should dress properly, be sensitive to the issues and needs, and have the proper manner in addressing the parents or family.

Working with an I/T

If using an I/T, the speech-language pathologist or audiologist should

1. provide extensive training to the I/T on the purposes, procedures, and goals of the tests and therapy methods. The I/T should also be taught to avoid the use of gestures, vocal intonation, and other cues that could inadvertently alert the individual to the correct response during the administration of tests.

2. preplan for an I/T's services to ensure that the individual understands the specific clinical procedures to be used.

3. use the same I/T(s) with a given language minority client rather than an I/T selected at random.

4. use client observation or other nonlinguistic measures as supplements to the translated measures, such as (a) the child's interaction with parents, (b) the child's interaction with peers, and (c) pragmatic analysis.

The speech-language pathologist and audiologist should state in the written evaluations that an I/T was used, as the validity of the results may be affected.

Clinicians who work with I/Ts must provide them with the best possible context for proper interpretation and translation. In giving the client information through an I/T, for example, the clinician should

- speak distinctly and at a normal pace.
- keep sentences short and simple.
- provide enough pauses for the I/T to organize his or her thoughts for proper translation.
- avoid excessive use of function words of items that can be difficult to translate.
- ask if the I/T needs clarification and elaboration.
- use abstract words sparingly. Words of feelings, attitudes, and qualities may not have the same meaning when translated directly. Because a direct translation may be misleading, a great deal of explanation may be required to convey the exact meaning.

Clinicians should avoid the use of certain types of expressions that cannot be easily translated. For example, literal translations of idioms do not carry the same meaning. English idioms such as *raining cats and dogs, give me a ring* (on the telephone), and *call him up,* and colloquial expressions such as *fat cat* and *pass the buck* have no equivalent in another language. Proverbs such as *the early bird catches the worm* may not be easily translated, and the I/T may not be familiar with the usage and meaning. Professional terminology and jargon, such as brain-stem evoked response, mesiocclusion, and phonology, may not have counterparts in another language; Furthermore, the I/T may not know what they mean. Similarly, complicated scoring results, such as standard score, z-scores, percentile ranks, and stanines, are difficult to translate and explain to the general audience.

It is important to establish rapport during an interview. The clinician should try to read the nonverbal cues from the listener and the I/T. If either looks puzzled, the clinician should try to explain in another way to clarify the message. Frequently, examples help to relax the I/T and to bring out the point more clearly. Most Asians nod their heads during an interview, giving the impression that they understand what is being said. Such a gesture is a matter of courtesy, however, and may not actually indicate that they understand the discussion. The clinician should check frequently to see if the interviewee understands by asking him or her to answer questions and provide examples. The clinician should always encourage feedback from the interviewee.

The clinician should keep the environment relaxed, nonthreatening, and comfortable. The I/T may be nervous, and it is important to set a relaxed tone while maintaining respect and proper distance. The clinician needs to be sensitive to the communication styles of the I/T and interviewee, keeping proximity at a comfortable distance and avoiding eye contact if it is too threatening to the Asian individuals. Finally, the clinician should check with the I/T periodically to make sure that he or she is not speaking too fast, too slowly, too softly, or unclearly and is not using too much jargon or unfamiliar words.

Although some parents are proficient in English, their communication style may interfere with true communication. In one instance, for example, a Laotian father attended a meeting to discuss an individualized education program (IEP) for his son. Throughout the meeting, the father nodded and said, "Yes," when the different participants in the meeting talked about their impression of the child and their recommendations. Finally, the father was asked whether he agreed with the placement and the recommendations. To everyone's surprise, he said, "No." Frustrated, the IEP team members did not understand why the father had continued to indicate "yes" when he did not agree with what was said. The father had nodded merely to indicate that he understood, however, not to indicate that he agreed. This behavior, however, caused a communication breakdown and resulted in misinterpretation.

In another case, bilateral neurosensory hearing loss was diagnosed in a 5-year-old Hmong boy with fluid in the middle ears. The school audiologist informed the father of the diagnosis and explained that the child needed to wear hearing aids and to take medication for otitis media. The father said, "Yes," when the audiologist asked him if he understood her. The audiologist felt uneasy about the session, however, and sought the help of a Hmong interpreter in the community. When the Hmong interpreter asked the father questions about the child's hearing problem, the father replied, "I don't know because I couldn't understand the lady [audiologist]." The Hmong interpreter then explained to the father about the child's hearing loss, the importance of the hearing aid, and the need for medication.

An I/T was also needed to help a 7-year-old Vietnamese girl who was described by her classroom teacher as a child who "cries easily, is not interested in learning, and has difficulty in verbal communication." The speech-language pathologist asked a bilingual resource teacher for help. When the Vietnamese-speaking teacher asked the child what was wrong, the child replied that she cried because she could not understand what the teacher wanted her to do and was too afraid of the teacher to ask questions. She was also afraid that whatever she did would not meet with the teacher's approval, so she cried from embarrassment. Although her speech was not clear, she could communicate effectively in Vietnamese. The speech-language pathologist tested the child's English articulation and found a number of substitutions; in addition, a vocabulary test revealed that the child's English vocabulary was below average. Thus, the child was having difficulty comprehending English and expressing herself in English. The child was referred for more training in English as a second language, and the classroom teacher began to explain things to her in a simple and repetitious manner. The child responded much better and stopped crying in class.

Role of the Bilingual Teacher and Aide

Rather than provide direct services to those students in need of speech and language services, the speech-language pathologist may work as a consultant in collaboration with a bilingual teacher and/or aide. Frassinelli, Superior, and Meyers (1983) pointed out that the consultation is a three-person chain of service in which (1) a consultant interacts with (2) a care-giver (consultee) to benefit (3) an individual (client) for whom the care-giver is responsible. A consultant provides professional services to the student indirectly through the teacher or the aide. There are certain advantages to the collaborative model:

1. The teacher and/or aide is with the child throughout the day and has ample opportunity to observe and interact with the child.

2. The child can remain in a language-learning situation during a greater part of the day, whereas a pull-out program for individual or group work is limited in contact time.
3. The teacher and/or aide speaks the native language of the child and, with training, can make judgments about the child's linguistic and communicative competence in his or her native language. Such information is extremely important to proper assessment.
4. With sufficient training, the teacher and/or aide may be able to identify potential speech, language, or hearing disorders that require follow-up intervention by a specialist.
5. Remediation of language disorders, which should be provided in the child's native language, can be incorporated into the everyday classroom activities (e.g., storytelling). With the assistance of the speech-language pathologist, the teacher can provide a program tailored for the child.

When there are no bilingual teachers and/or aides in the school, outside bilingual teachers and/or aides can be contracted and trained to assist in evaluation and remediation. Bilingual Asian school psychologists, anthropologists, linguists, special education teachers, resource teachers, social workers, and others working in a variety of settings may also be trained to work with the Asian LEP population in a team approach.

In addition, the training of bilingual teachers and/or aides should include information on

- universal language milestones
- language acquisition in primary languages
- second language acquisition
- cognitive and linguistic development of bilingual children (simultaneous and sequential)
- articulation screening
- language interference and transference
- techniques of collecting language samples
- contrastive analysis of phonology, morphology, and syntax
- basic analysis of language samples
- differences in cultures, semantics, and pragmatics
- observation in multiple contexts with multiple partners
- administration of bilingual tests

Role of Family Members and Friends

Family members may serve as informants and interactants in the assessment process. A child's interactions with his or her care-giver and siblings can be used for analysis of the child's communicative abilities. If the child says very little with the care-giver or sibling, the clinician should ask questions regarding the child's everyday interaction and behaviors. Older siblings without speech-language problems, as well as other Asian bilingual students in the school, may serve as informants and interactants.

Asian parents are often unaware of the expectations of school personnel and may themselves have very different expectations. Parents need to become familiar with the academic skills and discourse skills that their children need to succeed in school so they can assist their children at home. Cummins (1978) noted that basic interpersonal communication skills (BICS) differ from cognitive academic language proficiency (CALP) and that some children with good BICS have difficulty with CALP. Like Wong-Fillmore (1985) and Iglesias (1985), Cummins maintained that both skills are necessary for children to succeed in school. Speech-language clinicians need to examine both skills.

Community Resources

There are local associations for each of the Asian language minority groups, and the individual ethnic groups often operate language schools. For example, in 1986, there were 32 Chinese schools in New York and 104 Chinese schools in California (Lin, 1986). The teachers in the schools, as well as the organizers of the association, are good resources and can be used for the purposes of consultation, interpretation, interviews, and assistance in testing.

CHAPTER 8

The Assessment of Communicative Competence

A concept developed by Hymes (1971), communicative competence refers to an individual's ability to use language—perhaps best described as the ability to say the right thing in the right way at the right time in the right place. There are two major characteristics of communicative competence: (1) the ability to analyze the listener's role and (2) the ability to use linguistic resources in appropriate communication strategies. Studying communication and the acquisition of communicative competence from the functional view, Halliday (1978) concluded that the practice of learning language was the progressive development of a number of basic functions of language and the construction of meaning potentials.

Children's Acquisition of Communicative Competence

Children learn that the word *ball* means the object ball. Their knowledge about objects and events in the world comprises the content of their language. Children learn language-specific rules through continued exposure to the language and internal interpretation of the rules; English-speaking children, for example, learn to use the morpheme *-s* to indicate plurality and the morpheme *-ed* to indicate past tense. Their knowledge of pronunciation and grammar comprises the form of their language, while their knowledge of the function of language (e.g., to express feelings, to protest or comment, to request or deny) comprises the use of their language (Bloom & Lahey, 1978).

Most children acquire basic communicative competence by the age of 4 years without any formal teaching. They learn from their own experiences in their own environments in a natural way (Piaget, 1972; Uzgiris & Hunt, 1975). They learn to generate an infinite number of new sentences, most of which are appropriate for their communicative intents (Chomsky, 1965). Children from different language backgrounds learn different rules. By examining what competent communicators do in their language, researchers attempt to identify the different areas of knowledge that individuals must possess to attain communicative competence.

Halliday (1978) noted that a competent communicator must exhibit flexibility in many social contexts and roles, applying different rules to different situations. Since children have a limited vocabulary, they must convey many different communicative intents with only a small number of words. They may use the same form to convey different meanings (content) and serve entirely different functions. For example, young children may say "more" when they find more socks, "more" when they want more milk, and "more" when they ask for more cookies.

Slightly older children may experience other difficulties. Two different words often share the same meaning, but young children are limited in their semantic associations. For example, a child who had been asked to put something in the garbage can did not respond; when the garbage can was pointed out to him, he said, "That's not garbage can. That's trash can." Another child was asked to point to the picture of a magazine. She looked a little puzzled and then said, "I don't see a magazine. I see a Pennysaver [free classified advertisement flyer]."

Researchers and clinicians must examine the linguistic and nonlinguistic contexts closely and take into consideration interpersonal and intrapersonal functions of the language that children use in order to assess the children's communicative competence appropriately. Words and sentences are used in a certain way only because the people in a language community agree on such matters. These community norms, operations, principles, strategies, and interpretations support language comprehension (Smith, 1982). It is necessary to improve observation methods and to construct heuristically useful instruments to assess the abilities of children with limited English proficiency (LEP) and to evaluate their repertoires.

Linguistic and Cultural Differences

Simon (1979) created a framework for the study of communicative competence by dividing it into three major domains: form, function, and style (Table 8-1). This particular model, which presents both competent and incompetent features in communication, is based on the notion that it is necessary to examine children's communicative competence in order to assess their language skills. Many questions arise pertaining to the application of this clinical model, however. Certain features that Simon considered incompetent are not incompetent in the context of Asian culture. For example, a child's fear of asking adults questions, which Simon considered incompetent, is perceived as normal by Asian teachers and parents. Asian children are expected to be observant and quiet, speaking only in response to questions posed to them by adults. Furthermore, certain features that are considered incompetent in the mainstream model, such as difficulty with irregular verbs, plurals, and comparatives, are not relevant to some of the Asian languages.

Some LEP children exhibit good language abilities in their first language, but have difficulty expressing themselves in English. Many use ungrammatical sentences and structures in English that are awkward and incomprehensible to native speakers of English. Some LEP students do not comprehend English very well. Not every structure in one language has an equivalent in another language. For example, Bloom (1981) found that Chinese speakers had difficulty answering counterfactual questions:

> Judge: If you weren't leaving tomorrow, you would be deportable.
> Interpreter (*after struggling for an adequate translation*): I know you are leaving tomorrow, but if you do not leave, you will be deported.
> Taiwanese: But what do you mean? I am leaving tomorrow.
> (. . . *interpreter tries to convey the theoretical intent of the judge's statement; the Taiwanese persists in interpreting the judge's statement as a threat and in reiterating his intention of leaving . . .*)

Table 8-1 A Clinician's Model of Expressive Communicative Competence

Competent Features

Form	Function	Style
Flexible, precise vocabulary	Topics of conversation sustained	Consideration of listener's needs
Mastery of syntactic and morphological rules	Selected phrasing that reflects communicative intent	Advance planning of content
Complexity and variety of syntax	Provision of support for a point of view	Words easily found to express thoughts
Mastery of irregular grammatical features	Use of elaborated and restricted codes	Fluency in expression
Mastery of tense reference and subject/verb agreement	Social and cognitive uses of language	Intelligible, distinct speech
Use of clear noun referents	Development of heuristic language function	Comfortable speech rate
Use of subordinators to relate ideas	Contextual adaptations of language	Audible speech
	Tactful deviousness used	
	Modification and clarification of message upon listener request	

Incompetent Features

Form	Function	Style
Limited vocabulary repeated often	Wandering from conversational topic	Egocentric comments
Syntactic and morphological errors	Ineffective elocutionary speech acts	Incoherent sequencing of details
Basic syntactic patterns re-used	Opinions stated as fact	Difficulty in finding words
Difficulty with irregular verbs, plurals, and comparatives	Reliance on restricted code	False starts
Lack of consistency in tense and number reference	Informal, social uses of language	Slurred speech consisting of a series of "giant words"
Use of ambiguous pronouns	Fear of asking adults questions	Rapid, jerky speech rate
Unsystematic combinations of ideas	Limited language flexibility	Failure to adapt speech volume to context
	Tactless statements	
	Restatement of same information	

Source: From *Communicative Competence: A Functional-Pragmatic Approach to Language Therapy* (p. 3) by C. Simon, 1979, Tucson, Az.: Communication Skill Builders, Inc. Copyright 1979 by Communication Skill Builders, Inc. Reprinted by permission.

> Judge: If you have to be deported, where would you wish to be deported to?
> (*Taiwanese totally unable to comprehend;* . . . *finally interpreter counseled Taiwanese to respond: Taiwan*) (A. Bloom, 1981, p. 79)

In Chinese, there are no structures equivalent to those in English that mark the counterfactual realm. Consequently, when presented with questions that contain a counterfactual hypothesis, Chinese speakers fail to comprehend the communicative intent of the speaker. Such a situation often leads to confusion and communication breakdowns.

Syntax. Basic information on the syntax of the first language may help the clinician understand the incorrect word order that Asian students sometimes use in English. Also, since most of the Asian languages are not inflectional,

Asian LEP students frequently omit verb tense markers, plural markers, and gender markers. With practice, however, Asian students can generally master the use of these markers in English.

Semantics. Words are learned in context. The same word may have different meanings, depending on the context and the intent of the speaker. In English, for example, the word *sharp* in the knife is *sharp*, she is a *sharp*-looking girl, and she is *sharp* has three different meanings. In the last case, the word *sharp* implies intelligent; however, the same *sharp* in Chinese means *cunning*—in a pejorative sense.

Receptive Vocabulary. Clinicians generally use pictures to test children's receptive vocabulary. The clinician names an item and asks the child to point to the correct picture. This procedure gives the clinician a sense of the child's receptive vocabulary. Although a Picture Vocabulary Test can be used to obtain a baseline of an Asian child's English vocabulary, the clinician must take care to remove (1) those culturally biased items that are unfamiliar to most Asian language minorities, (2) those that cannot be translated to represent the same degree of linguistic complexity, (3) those that have no equivalent in the native language of the child, and (4) those that can be translated only by using two or more words of the child's native language. When such items have been removed, the clinician must adjust the score and modify its interpretation. With these adjustments, the results obtained should be considered an extremely crude estimate of the child's overall receptive vocabulary.

Tempo. Speech-language clinicians must pay attention not only to the forms of language, but also to the voice quality in which the messages are transmitted. Researchers in voice quality of American English speakers (e.g., Bowling, 1980) have reported that Americans often consider individuals who speak at a rapid rate to be untrustworthy and individuals who speak at a slow rate to be stupid. In contrast, Asians consider those who speak rapidly to be efficient, sharp, and impatient, while they consider those who speak slowly to be well-mannered, lucid, and stable. Perceptions of pitch and vocal intensity may also vary.

Intensity. The model developed by Simon (1979) points to certain verbal styles as incompetent, for example, failure to adapt speech volume to context. Again, the volume of speech is determined in large part by the cultural context in which conversation takes place. The following illustrates a Chinese schoolgirl's attitude toward her voice:

> When my second grade class did a play, the whole class went to the auditorium except the Chinese girls. The teacher, lovely and Hawaiian, should have understood about us, but instead left us behind in the classroom. Our voices were too soft or nonexistent, and our parents never signed the permission slips anyway. They never signed anything unnecessary.

It is customary for Japanese executives to use low-pitched voices of very low intensity to indicate power and authority. This is not considered incompetent in Japan. Similar vocal qualities in U.S. executives may be interpreted as a lack of confidence, however.

Because of the differences among languages and cultures, a model of communicative competence must be constructed for each language minority. Clinicians must become cross-culturally competent in order to obtain valid assessments of children's language abilities. Consequently, it is necessary to adapt the mainstream model to ensure that it is suitable and appropriate for clinicians who work with the Asian multicultural population.

Holistic Approach to Assessment

Research in the sociolinguistic tradition has indicated that the study of communication in a naturalistic or natural context facilitates the assessment of communicative competence. In the assessment of a child's communicative competence, therefore, clinicians should view communication as an interactive and dynamic process by addressing the following questions:

1. How competent is the child in communication in his or her native language?
2. How competent is the child in communication in his or her second language?
3. How does the child use his or her language or languages?
4. What purposes do the child's communications serve?
5. Is the child successful in expressing his or her needs?
6. Are the child's needs met?
7. How is the flow of communication between the child and his or her parents? between the child and his or her siblings? between the child and his or her peers? between the child and his or her teachers?
8. What kind of communication breakdowns does the child present?
9. Are these breakdowns typically problems that are caused by differences in culture?
10. Does the child have a language problem in his or her native language?
11. What are these problems?
12. What are the possible causes for the problems?
13. What is the child capable of communicating?
14. Are there other factors that should be taken into consideration?

Ethnographic Approach

Ethnography is a method of studying events and people that takes into account the underlying rules that operate for the study participants. In recent years, there has been an increasing interest in the application of ethnographic techniques to the study of education and the learning process. Some researchers, such as Heath (1983), Wong-Fillmore (1985), Gumperz (1982), and Philips (1983), have concentrated their efforts on the ethnography of communication. They have studied communicative processes and attempted to determine the meaning of communicative interaction by analyzing linguistic, paralinguistic, nonlinguistic, sociocultural, and contextual aspects of the communicative act. They have advocated a holistic sociocultural approach to the study of communication. In addition, they have agreed that the core of the study of communication is communicative competence. Cook-Gumperz and Gumperz (1979) stated:

> We should no more attempt to measure communicative competence than we should attempt to devise a single test that will capture everything. . . . Rather than use communicative competence as a basis to devise tests of language competence, this concept is better used as a diagnostic notion to sharpen and focus the basic qualitative tools of ethnography. Its value lies in its potential for deepening our understanding of the complexities involved, and ensuring the transmission of knowledge as a process of conversational experience and communicative understanding. (p.21)

They stated further that

> we consider the teacher to be in a position as an everyday ethnographer of education.

Communicative acts can be explored through looking at participant structures which are the norms of participation . . . in governing the type and quantity of interaction that make the event. (p. 21)

Inadequacies of Instrumentation

Although some assessment instruments include pragmatics, most are consistent with the traditional approach of collecting results from linguistically oriented tests for the assessment of communicative competence. Nevertheless, there is a recognized need to emphasize sociocultural and cognitive knowledge, as well as pragmatics, in the examination of children. Ethnographic methodology incorporates all of these areas. In recent years, several language researchers (Kayser, 1986; Ripich & Spinelli, 1985; Wilkinson, 1982) have begun to utilize it. Noting the lack of instruments for assessing and measuring individual communicative competence, Dickson (1982) stated, "Neither the socio-linguistic nor the referential tradition has produced instruments suitable . . . to assess children's communicative competence" (p. 134). In the area of multicultural assessment, instruments are even more scarce.

It is necessary to develop an instrument that will provide clinicians and teachers with a protocol to determine what children know and can do as communicators. The construction of such an instrument should allow for individual differences in communicative competence and in cultural background. The difficulties of organizing such a set of techniques for assessing children's communicative competence are enormous. In the past, a few assessment instruments have been designed in which referential communicative performance is used to assess communicative competence in a more natural setting (Aaronson & Schaefer, 1971; Cazden 1972; Chandler, Greenspan, & Barenboim, 1974). No standardized instruments have been developed, however. Standardized test batteries measure context-free skills, but communication is context-bound and content-specific.

When there are incongruencies in communication styles and expectations between customary norms of their native culture and those of the less familiar mainstream American culture, children tend to experience confusion and conflicts and to retain the older, more familiar patterns. In order to achieve a more accurate assessment of an individual child's communicative competence, clinicians must adopt a technique that encompasses the effects of that child's cultural background.

Micro-Ethnographic Approach

The use of micro-ethnography through systematic observation can reveal much about the natural language functioning of children, that is, their language use and communication in specific contexts (Erickson, 1978). According to Trueba and Wright (1980-81), micro-ethnographers systematically search for specific events, using sophisticated taping methods; do discourse analysis; redefine holism in terms of structural cohesiveness; interrelate segments of an interactional act; and attempt to make sense of what they observe by grounding the inferences in the specifics of the observed behavior. The focus of micro-ethnographic study is the quality of interaction, as well as the quantity of events (Ripich & Spinelli, 1985). Micro-ethnographic methods can be used to examine children's communicative acts with multiple partners in multiple/naturalistic environments.

Many researchers have advocated the use of naturalistic assessment with monolingual English-speaking children (Lund & Duchan, 1983; Prizant, 1978). According to Wilson (1977), two hypotheses comprise the rationale for micro-ethnographic methods. First—the naturalistic ecological hypothesis—it is essential to study events in their natural setting in order to observe contextual influences. Second—the qualitative difference hypothesis—it is essential to study nonlinguistic and paralinguistic features of communication, as they *may* be culturally bound. Children who have language difficulties often exhibit nonverbal characteristics, such as a low frustration threshold or a short attention span, that create communication breakdowns. The evaluator may misinterpret such behaviors as evidence of a communicative disorder. Thus, it is extremely helpful to observe how well children communicate with speakers of their native language, within the framework of ongoing interactions rather than to focus on the end product (i.e., speech phenomenon) alone.

Ethnographic research places great emphasis on examining interactions, frame by frame, in order to gain a holistic picture of the communication act. Hymes (1974) described the approach as follows:

1. As to scope of language study, one cannot take separate results from linguistics, psychology, sociology, ethnology, and seek to correlate them. If one is to have a theory of language, one needs fresh kinds of data to investigate directly the use of language in context, as to discern patterns proper to speech patterns that escaped separate studies.
2. As to basis, one cannot take linguistic form, a given code or even speech itself, as a limiting frame of reference. One must take as context, a community or network of persons, investigating its communicative activities as a whole, so that any use of channel and code takes its place as part of the resources upon which the members draw. (pp. 3–4)

The importance of looking at the communication act as a whole was clearly emphasized by Halliday (1975), who believed that children must construct a system of meaning that represents their own model of reality. This process is a cognitive one that occurs in a particular sociocultural community. When assessing a child's communicative abilities, therefore, it is imperative to provide a natural/naturalistic social context that allows interactions to be more realistic and to reflect more accurately the child's actual capabilities. Ripich and Spinelli (1985) proposed the following framework:

Step 1. Identify the child.
Step 2. Describe the communication breakdown.
Step 3. Develop a summary of problems.
Step 4. Observe the interaction in the classroom.
Step 5. Summarize observations and identify patterns of communication breakdowns.
Step 6. Validate observation.

Clinicians who work with the Asian multicultural population group need to use this type of framework if the assessment is to reflect the children's communication/language competencies without misinterpretation or inaccuracies based on the clinicians' cultural/language bias.

Exhibit 8-1 Ethrographic Assessment of Children's Communicative Competence

Concepts

The Assessment of Children's Communicative Competence / Communicative Competence / Name: / Age: / Responses	1. Unintelligible response	2. No response	3. Verbal	4. Nonverbal	5. Vocal	6. Repeat	7. Label	8. Request	9. Demand	10. Comment	11. Imitation	12. Response to wh-question	13. Greeting	14. Description of object act	15. Answering questions	16. Asking question	17. Expressing need	18. Description of event	19. Description of own act	20. Description of past experience	21. Description of plan	22. Description of photo, picture	23. Topic initiation	24. Topic shift	25. Off-topic response	26. Topic maintenance
Total																											

In the assessment of Asian children's communicative competence, a holistic/naturalistic/experiental approach may be used to perform an in-depth analysis of the communication between the children and their interactants, especially their classroom teacher, aides, resource teachers, siblings, parents, and peers. This approach, best described as an ethnographic approach to assessment based on the constructivist view, focuses on extensive descriptive and interpretative efforts and the explanation of complex behaviors. Clinicians not only observe naturalistic interactions in contexts familiar to the child, but also provide challenging situations that are unfamiliar to the child.

The interview technique facilitates interaction. When necessary, the clinician can create specific contexts, for example, by asking the child to describe the procedure used to make something or to describe a photograph. The instrument shown in Exhibit 8-1 takes into consideration the importance of multiple descriptions in a number of contexts and the need to determine the child's abilities in both his or her native language and in English. The instrument requires careful observation of the child's reactions and responses in a variety of contexts, and the clinician should have a background in ethnography before using it. The child's responses are recorded verbatim on the left-hand side of the instrument. Each response is evaluated based on the categories numbered 1 to 26 listed at the top of the instrument. The number of responses in each category is tallied and the total is entered at the bottom of the grid. A blank category indicates a lack of response in that area. The total responses in a particular category reflects the ability to use that category. The overall variety of the child's responses is indicated by the number of categories used.

Through careful analysis of the information on this ethnographic assessment instrument, the clinician can determine how Asian LEP students use language and what materials will be interesting, motivating, and meaningful to them. With its emphasis on the domain of pragmatics, this instrument may be used to study children who do poorly on standardized tests. The findings of such an interactional analysis can reveal important data that can not be obtained by using any standardized testing procedure, especially when the children tested do not understand or respond to the test. It is through naturalistic observation and interaction that the teacher and the speech-language pathologist learn about children and their use of language.

CHAPTER 9

Assessment Procedures

The goal of language assessment is to obtain information about an individual's communicative competence. Since all children learn to talk and communicate, it is the children's past experiences, their culture, and their environment that makes the difference in the way that they use language. The use of a naturalistic approach to assessment may reveal previously unrecognized communicative competence in language minority children. When provided with an experiential, facilitative, and naturalistic context (together with a testing environment that stimulates exploration, rather than restricts and controls activities), these children will respond differently, interact more readily, create more abundantly, and communicate more effectively.

Assessment of the communicative abilities of a child should take place in naturalistic environments that decrease anxiety and increase motivation. The clinician should attempt to create assessment procedures that are culturally and pragmatically appropriate. For example, the clinician might:

- ask the child to relate an event or an incident
- ask the child to tell a story if story-telling is part of the family routine
- show the child a picture and ask him or her to tell a story about the picture
- ask the child to choose a game and to explain how the game is played (if the child is familiar with the game)
- create new games with the child
- ask the child to teach another child or a group of children how to play a game or how to make something
- work with the child on a small project (e.g., making birthday decorations) and, after the project has been completed, ask the child to describe the things required to complete the project and the sequence of events from beginning to end
- ask the child to bring something from home and to talk about it

Detailed information on the child's background and past experiences is most helpful in finding activities that are not only stimulating to the child, but also permit an accurate evaluation of the cognitive development of the child.

Clark (1984) reported that children spend only 18% of their time in school. That which they learn outside the school, in the community and at home, contributes significantly to the way in which they understand concepts, structure and classify them, analyze and synthesize them, store and retrieve them, and generate their own concepts in oral or written forms. Because these forms are meaningful and have been learned through their past experiences, the ability to talk about these past experiences is very important. Therefore, the clinician may ask parents to bring photograph albums, books, objects, and toys from home, pictures of activities and events, such as birthday parties or trips to the zoo, which may be used later to elicit descriptions.

By involving parents in the assessment process, clinicians are able to gain insight into the most appropriate assessment procedures for the children.

Nonbiased Assessment

At the present time, educators have the enormous responsibility of providing an assessment that is linguistically, culturally, cognitively, and socially meaningful to Asian language minorities. The need for culturally nonbiased testing has made both professionals and researchers take a close look at the existing assessment instruments to determine their possible bias (Baca & Cervantes, 1984; Oller, 1978; Omark & Erickson, 1983). They assert that if children, for example, cannot make sense of the task given because of their social, cultural, and linguistic differences as well as their learning and cognitive styles, their abilities cannot be appropriately assessed (Anderson, 1987).

The dilemmas that educators face in the assessment of Asian children's language abilities are complex and difficult to solve because the process of language acquisition is very complicated and because current understanding of the distinction between the different and the disordered is incomplete. The use of ethnographic methods in the observation and description of Asian language minority children's communication in both their native language and in English has revealed that there is an enormous range and a great diversity of language differences among them. By the same token, monolingual children also exhibit an enormous range and diversity in their communicative behaviors.

In testing children from language minority backgrounds, care must be taken to ensure that the items used are familiar to the children. The following is a list of some elements that may be unfamiliar to Asian language minority children in tests:

- household objects: items for baking (as most Asians are unfamiliar with baking and the use of an oven); certain cooking utensils; furniture items; spreads, comforters, and fitted sheets
- vehicles: trains, cable car, ambulance, police car, garbage truck, cleaning truck, even a school bus
- sports: football, hockey, tobogganing, skiing, sky-diving, surfing, wind-surfing, archery, water-skiing, camping
- musical instruments: drums, guitar, banjo, harmonica, piano, accordion
- clothing: tie, suspenders, slips, underwear, raincoat, boots, galoshes, mittens, gloves, hats, slippers
- professionals: doctor, judge, firefighter
- buildings and signs: danger signs, traffic signs, ranches, bungalows, gazebo, baseball diamond, garbage cans, mailbox
- historically related events and people: Thanksgiving, George Washington, Abraham Lincoln, pioneer, Daniel Boone, astronaut, past presidents

- commercial items and famous people and figures: Mickey Mouse, Superman, He-Man
- historically related items and buildings: the Statue of Liberty, the Liberty Bell, the White House, the Capitol
- holidays and activities associated with them: Christmas, Halloween, Easter, Easter eggs, valentines
- foods: pumpkin pie, apple pie, yogurt
- school-related events: homecoming, initiation, proms, Parent-Teacher Association
- customs: baby showers, wedding showers
- values represented by stories: bravery, honesty, respect
- geography: New York, Chicago, Seattle, Great Lakes
- community activities: camp, Boy Scouts
- children's programs: *Sesame Street, Mr. Roger's Neighborhood*
- brand names: Kleenex, Xerox
- games: hopscotch, hide and seek, tag, Monopoly
- nursery rhymes: Jack and Jill, Little Jack Horner
- children's stories and folklore: Three Little Pigs, Little Red Riding Hood, The Three Bears

Potentially biased elements should be noted when results are recorded and analyzed. Erikson and Iglesias (1986) provided guidelines for adapting standardized instruments for assessing the language minority population. These included going beyond the list, asking the child to explain why he or she incorrectly chose an item, and asking the child to name rather than point to an item.

A Cognitive-Ecological-Functional Model for Assessment

Combining observations of cognitive strategies required by the various ecological settings in which communication occurs and of the different functions of language, facilitates the evaluation of a child's communicative competence. This cognitive-ecological-functional model takes into account the fact that a child often behaves differently in different ecological settings. Given cognitively demanding tasks, the model provides the clinician with insight into the child's problem-solving and communicative abilities. Given multiple ecological settings with multiple partners at various levels, the model provides clinicians and observers with the opportunity to investigate the child's language function. The assessment procedure is presented in a checklist format with four major areas: (1) information gathering, (2) consultation/conference, (3) systematic observation, and (4) assessment of communicative abilities. See Appendix A for the protocol of the instrument described below.

Information Gathering (See Item 1, Appendix A, p. 161.)

The most essential process in the assessment of an individual's speech, language, and hearing skills is information gathering. Asian language minority individuals referred to speech-language pathologists have a wide range of communicative competence in English. They may speak no English, limited English, or fluent English. Their backgrounds are so culturally and linguistically diverse that clinicians must first of all obtain a thorough history, including medical history, family history, previous education, immigration history (refugee, illegal alien, or landed immigrant), the time of arrival in the United States, intervening experiences, the number of years in the United States, home language(s), psychological or adjustment history. With the help of a trained interpreter/translator, if necessary, speech-language pathologists may obtain such vital information by using questionnaires and structured interviews (Appendixes B through E).

School work and records both from previous schools and from current schools yield valuable information about a child's overall learning patterns and behaviors. A medical history and a development history are essential in the pre-assessment information-gathering process. Reports on the child's participation in any English as a second language (ESL) program can provide valuable information about the child's second language acquisition.

Care must be taken to examine the reason for a referral, and a medical examination that includes an evaluation of hearing, vision, and motor function is recommended at this time. Medical intervention may be indicated after the examination. On occasion, psychological evaluation and counseling may be warranted.

Consultation/Conference (See Item 2, Appendix A, p. 161.)

Speech-language clinicians can obtain substantial information about Asian language minority children by consulting with individuals who have special knowledge about their behaviors and performance. For example, the classroom teacher can provide valuable information about a child's rate of learning and learning style, personal relational style, cognitive style, and classroom behavior. The classroom teacher has the opportunity to observe the child in multiple contexts, such as reading, show and tell, sharing, group assignments, group projects, and individual desk work. Similarly, resource teachers can provide information about the child's performance in any special program in which he or she may be enrolled. Furthermore, resource teachers can provide information and materials about the child's first language.

Students of limited English proficiency (LEP) typically receive training in ESL when they begin school. Teachers in the ESL program can compare the child's progress in ESL class with that of other children in the class. Frequently, the LEP child who is referred for assessment began ESL training at the same time that his or her siblings began the training. Thus, the ESL teacher can compare the child's performance to that of the siblings, who have usually been exposed to similar linguistic/social/cultural environments.

School psychologists are most helpful in providing information about the language minority child's cognitive style, social adaptive skills, attention, etc. They have often assessed the child using informal measures as well as nonverbal performance tests, and the information may help the speech-language clinician to determine which assessment strategies are most appropriate for the child. Other school personnel, such as the school nurse, the social worker, the teaching aides, and the students who can speak the child's first language, can provide information about the child's home language, home culture, and cognitive/linguistic skills.

The parents of the child can provide very valuable information about the child's performance and language skills, as they can judge the communicative competence of the child at home and in the community. Furthermore, the parents can provide historical data on the child's acquisition of the first language, as well as comparative data on the language skills of the child, other children at home, and other children in the community. Other native speakers of the child's first language can also judge the child's communicative competence in that language.

Systematic Observation (*See Item 3, Appendix A, p. 161.*)

Children can be observed with many different people in many places, such as in school, in the classroom, at home, or on the playground. Observation in these multiple settings makes it possible to obtain information about the child's overall communication behaviors in multiple contexts. Furthermore, the multiple inter-actants can serve as informants about the child's speech and language abilities. A home visit is a requirement. If it is not feasible, a parent interview is a must.

In observing LEP students, clinicians and educators should determine what the students know and do not know, what they like and do not like, and what motivates them and does not motivate them. The clinician may provide them with a variety of toys or books, or may ask them to bring their favorite toys or play objects, or anything they want to share from home. The clinician should watch them interact with peers, teachers, aides, siblings, parents, and even strangers. All communicative attempts whether verbal, nonverbal, vocal, intelligible, unintelligible, responsive, or nonresponsive, should be recorded.

Children have a wide range of cognitive learning and behavioral styles, as well as communicative, personal, and relational styles, many of which can be attributed to cultural differences. The clinician who is assessing the communicative abilities of children must take into consideration the commonalities of the communicative process, however. For example, all children learn to label things, and all children learn to talk about their needs. Some may have had more experience with "naming drills," than others. Moreover, observing children's interactions with multiple partners may provide the clinician with an impression of the flexibility of their communicative style as they adjust to the different interactants. The clinician needs to obtain from multiple informants their impressions of the child through systematic observation. These informal observations include:

- motivation
- attention
- concentration
- emotion
- organization
- sequencing
- problem solving
- repetition
- social behavior
- adjustment
- giving directions
- following directions
- giving responses
- asking questions
- using clarification or emphasis
- applicant's exit from text

In order to observe children's problem-solving skills, the clinician may suggest that the children imagine certain situations. These might include such differing situations as:

- The door is locked.
- The room is dark.
- The drapes are drawn.
- The tape recorder is not plugged in.
- The floor is dirty.
- The lid on the jar is too tight.
- A piece of the puzzle is missing.
- A part of a toy is missing.
- The toy cannot be reached.
- The table is dirty or messy.
- The chair is on the floor.
- The chair is missing.
- The table is wet.

Other techniques that may facilitate interactions include

- hiding objects in bags and containers and asking the child to find them
- concealing objects from the children and asking them to find them
- presenting objects with missing parts
- presenting children with novel, unfamiliar objects
- engaging children in role-plays
- presenting pictures of familiar or unfamiliar objects and asking them to comment
- creating disruptions in the act of play
- asking children questions (e.g., wh- questions)
- asking children to demonstrate and tell about a prescribed sequence of behavior (e.g., making a hamburger out of clay)
- eliciting schemas and scripts (e.g., have you been to McDonald's? What did you have at McDonald's?)
- asking them to carry out simple commands or a sequence of commands
- playing different kinds of games
- asking them to complete a sequence of activities (e.g., cutting out pictures and putting them in a scrapbook) when not all the necessary items are immediately at hand (e.g., no glue on the table), thus making the task cognitively demanding

A checklist can be helpful in assessing the communicative abilities of Asian LEP students (Appendix F). It is also helpful to use a behavioral observation checklist to identify the problem area(s) in a student's communication (Appendix G). The clinician, as well as teachers, must be aware of the many factors that influence the success or failure of an interaction.

It is necessary to examine the assessment instruments used with Asian LEP students, to sharpen the available analytical tools, to conduct research on these students, and to examine the policies and practices in assessing their language proficiency. There is a need for clinicians to improve observational methods, to examine communicative competence in various contexts, to analyze a large piece of discourse, and to determine how Asian LEP students sequence events, organize ideas, acquire information through incidental learning, react to pressure, express abstract thinking, make inferences, and store and retrieve networks of information. Clinicians must recognize the limitations of quantitative analysis and conduct ethnographic studies that will permit improvement in assessment procedures for Asian LEP children.

Assessment of Communicative Abilities (*See Item 4, Appendix A, p. 162.*)

In assessing the English competence of Asian LEP students, the clinician may use (1) vocabulary tests to obtain an estimate of their expressive/receptive one word repertoire, (2) tests of auditory comprehension to determine their level of comprehension, (3) stories to obtain a language sample from the students, and (4) articulation tests and stimulability tests (providing stimulus items for a child to imitate or repeat) to obtain an inventory of their articulation. (See Appendix H for sample tests for Mandarin and Vietnamese.) Many Asian children are not familiar with the turn-taking strategies in oral language interactions and may find taking tests intimidating. Because Asians generally encourage their children to keep quiet unless they are spoken to, the clinician may find questionnaires useful to initiate the assessment session and to establish a rapport with these children. Although some may not test well, they are capable of answering questions in natural settings.

In terms of pragmatics, speech-language clinicians must understand that pragmatic rules are culturally bound and context specific. The Peanut Butter Test (Craighead, 1987) is a test of pragmatics that has been found useful in working with American children. Test items include requests for assistance, asking questions, etc. In examining the items on the test, one may find many items culturally inappropriate for adaptation for Asian populations, since most Asian children out of respect will probably not ask the teacher any questions. Based on the Peanut Butter Test, selected items might be helpful in assessing the pragmatic rules of the Asian children.

In those children who are experiencing difficulty in school, it may be necessary to evaluate reading and writing abilities. Speech-language clinicians must find out whether the LEP children were literate in their native language before their immigration to the United States. If not, testing in English will reveal important information about their English literacy skills.

With the assistance of multiple informants, monolingual speech-language clinicians can obtain a substantial amount of information about the Asian LEP students' abilities in their first language by determining whether the students

	Adequate	Questionable
1. use labels		
2. use simple declarative sentences		
3. use question forms		
4. describe past, present, and future events		
5. use prepositions		
6. use adjectives		
7. use comparatives		
8. use colors		
9. name body parts		
10. use request, command, protest		
11. use negation		
12. count sequentially		

	Adequate	Questionable
13. use numerals	_____	_____
14. use pronouns	_____	_____
15. use commentaries	_____	_____
16. distinguish singularity from plurality	_____	_____
17. use native language sound system	_____	_____

Pictures and objects can be used to elicit labels, action words, adjectives, pronouns, comparatives, colors, numerals, body parts, and prepositions, both in native language and English (Appendix I).

Narratives (See Item 4, Appendix A, p. 162.)

Stories from a child's own cultural background facilitate the assessment of the child's ability to use the accounting (i.e., description of a present event), recounting (i.e., description of a past event) and eventcasting (i.e., description of a future event) functions of language. In a story-telling activity the child may be able to use all three functions. Questions such as the following may be useful:

- What happened to the little boy?
- What do you think will happen?
- What do you think the little girl is going to do?
- Do you remember what happened to the little boy?
- What is the rabbit doing now?

Stories in English may be adapted to make them culturally appropriate and relevant to Asian language minority children (Appendix J).

Many themes for stories are culture-fair. For example, all caterpillars turn into butterflies, and all tadpoles turn into frogs. When the sunlight shines on raindrops, a rainbow appears in the sky. All children know about the sun, the moon, the stars, the sunset, and the sunrise. Commonly occurring themes that involve foods, animals, plants, flowers, people, colors, shapes, numbers, weather, clothing, housing, family, and places are good material for culture-fair stories. Furthermore, unfamiliar items can be used and introduced in stories so that they can be rechecked later for retention. For example, a story of a child with freckles (most Asians don't have freckles) can be introduced in one session and rechecked in a later one. These stories can be used to assess children's skills in both their native language and English (Appendix J).

Cloze Test (See Item 4, Appendix A, p. 162.)

Clinicians may use a Cloze test which was introduced by Oller (1979) to obtain information about a child's level of comprehension, as well as level of expression, both in the child's native language and in English if the child can understand some English. The test can be given in written form or in oral form for those who cannot read. The key to the successful use of Cloze tests is the selection of materials appropriate for the culture and age of the child. In this instance, the term *age* refers to the child's *language* age rather than chronological age. For example, a 12-year-old boy who has been in the United States for only a few months may need materials in English suitable for children much younger than he; however, materials for a Cloze test in his native language should be appropriate for his chronological age.

Materials written in the native language of Asian LEP children, such as popular stories from their native country, can be used for a Cloze test. Bilingual resource teachers are generally very helpful in obtaining suitable materials. As Oller noted, the text should present material that is culturally relevant or has already been used in the child's class. Disturbing topics should be avoided. Because the test should contain at least 50 items, the text should be 250–350 words in length (if every fifth, sixth, or seventh word is to be deleted). The clinician can create multiple forms of the test from the same material by beginning to count deletions at a different point (e.g., starting at the third word rather than the first word).

In administering the test, the clinician may give these instructions:

> In the following passage, some of the words have been left out. First, read over the entire passage and try to understand what it is about. Then, try to fill in the blanks. It takes exactly one word to fill in each blank. . . . If you are not sure of the word that has been left out, guess. (Oller, 1979, p. 366)

The clinician may present an example:

> The _____ barked furiously, and the _____ ran up the tree.
> The words that correctly fill in the blanks are *dog* and *cat*.

Examples may be given in the child's native language. For young children, the instructions should be simplified.

In presenting the test orally for a nonreader, the clinician should (1) read the text aloud two or three times, (2) question the child about the story to be sure that the child comprehends the subject matter, and (3) read the story aloud again, asking the child to supply missing words. If the child cannot supply the missing word, the clinician goes back to the beginning of the sentence and reads forward to the next missing word.

A Cloze test may be scored on the basis of either "exact words" (i.e., the words that were used in the original text) or "contextually appropriate words" (i.e., words that fit the sentences). Each method provides a range of scores, and each produces the same distribution of high and low scorers (Oller, 1979). The clinician may examine the particular errors made by students to develop instructional programs in language remediation. Students should pass at least half of the items *in English* before taking an English language test (whether verbal or nonverbal). It should be noted that these techniques have now been used with equal success for Czech, English, French, German, Japanese, Polish, Swedish, Thai, and Vietnamese individuals.

The following example of Cloze test material is taken from a book entitled *Popular Stories from Vietnam*.

The Most Pleasant and Unpleasant Thing in the Whole World

> Once there was a rich man who had a clever cook. One day the man called his cook and said, "You have cooked many kinds of food for me. I like them very much. Today I want to taste the most pleasant thing in the world. Please buy it and cook it for me."
> The cook went to the market. But he could not decide what the most pleasant thing in the world was. He thought very hard for a few minutes. Then he smiled. He went quickly to the meat shop, bought the tongue* of a pig and went back to the house.

---

*A tongue = the part in the middle of the mouth. It has no bone and it moves when people talk. A person cannot talk without a tongue.

After he cooked the tongue, he brought it to the man and said, "Sir, you asked me to cook the most pleasant thing in the world. Here it is."

The man was very surprised when he saw the tongue of a pig. He asked the cook why he thought the tongue was the most pleasant thing in the world. The cook answered quickly, "Sir, when people love each other, their tongues say the most pleasant things to each other. Is the tongue not the most pleasant thing in the whole world?"

The man thought that the cook's answer was very clever. A few days later, the man called his cook again and said, "Now I want to taste the most unpleasant thing in the world. Please buy it and cook it for me."

The cook went to the market quickly. He did not have to think very hard this time. He went straight to the butcher's shop and again bought the tongue of a pig. He went home, cooked it and brought it to the man and said, "Sir, this is the most unpleasant thing in the world."

The man was more surprised than before when he saw the tongue of a pig again. He asked the cook why he thought the tongue was the most unpleasant thing in the world this time. The cook answered, "Sir, when people hate each other, their tongues say the most unpleasant things to each other. Is the tongue not the most unpleasant thing in the whole world?"*

The Most Pleasant and Unpleasant Thing in the Whole World

Once there was a rich man _____ had a clever cook. One day _____ man called his cook and said, "You have _____ many kinds of food for me. I _____ them very much. Today I want to _____ the most pleasant thing in the _____. Please buy it and cook it for _____."

The cook went to the _____. But he could not decide what the _____ pleasant thing in the world _____. He thought very hard for a _____ minutes. Then he smiled. He went quickly to the _____ shop, bought the tongue† of a _____ and went back to the _____.

After he cooked the _____, he brought it to the _____ and said, "Sir, you asked me to _____ the most pleasant thing in the _____. Here it is."

The man was very _____ when he saw the tongue of a pig. He asked the cook _____ he thought the tongue was the most _____ thing in the world. The cook answered _____, "Sir, when people love each _____, their tongues say the most _____ things to each other. Is the tongue not the _____ pleasant thing in the whole world?"

The _____ thought that the cook's answer was very _____. A few days later, the man _____ his cook again and said, "Now I want to _____ the most unpleasant _____ in the world. Please buy it and cook it for _____."

The cook went to the _____ quickly. He did not have to think very _____ this time. He went straight to the _____ shop and again bought the _____ of a pig. He went home, cooked it and brought _____ to the man and said, "Sir, this is the _____ unpleasant thing in the world."

The man was more _____ than before when he saw the _____ of a pig again. He asked the _____ why he thought the tongue was the most _____ thing in the world this time. The cook answered, "_____, when people hate each other, their _____ say the most unpleasant things to each _____. Is the tongue not the most unpleasant _____ in the whole world?"

---

* From *Popular Stories from Vietnam* (pp. 29-34) by The Institute for Cultural Pluralism, San Diego: San Diego State University.

† A tongue=the part in the middle of the mouth. It has no bone and it moves when people talk. A person cannot talk without a tongue.

The following version of the same story—in Vietnamese—can be used to pre-pare a Cloze test for the child who is a native speaker of Vietnamese.

VẬT NGON NHỨT VÀ DỞ NHỨT TRÊN ĐỜI

NGÀY XƯA, CÓ MỘT ÔNG PHÚ-HỘ* NUÔI MỘT NGƯỜI ĐẦU BẾP THẬT KHÔN NGOAN. NGÀY KIA ÔNG PHÚ-HỘ GỌI NGƯỜI ĐẦU BẾP LÊN VÀ BẢO, "ANH ĐÃ NẤU CHO TA* NHIỀU MÓN ĂN RỒI. TA RẤT HÀI LÒNG. HÔM NAY TA MUỐN NẾM THỬ MỘT MÓN ĂN NGON NHỨT TRÊN ĐỜI NÀY. ANH LÀM ƠN ĐI MUA VỀ NẤU CHO TA ĂN XEM NÀO."

NGƯỜI ĐẦU BẾP ĐI RA CHỢ NHƯNG KHÔNG BIẾT CHỌN MÓN GÌ LÀ NGON NHỨT. SAU MỘT LÁT SUY NGHĨ ANH TA MỈM CƯỜI VÌ ĐÃ TÌM ĐƯỢC KẾ. ANH VỘI VÀNG ĐI LẠI HÀNG THỊT TÌM MUA MỘT CÁI LƯỠI CON HEO ĐEM VỀ.

SAU KHI NẤU XONG ANH TA DỌN LÊN CHO CHỦ ĂN VÀ THƯA, "THƯA ÔNG, ĐÂY LÀ MÓN NGON NHỨT TRÊN ĐỜI NÀY".

NGƯỜI PHÚ HỘ NGẠC NHIÊN VÔ CÙNG KHI THẤY

*phú-hộ: người giàu có (a rich man)
*ta: kẻ trên xưng với kẻ dưới, nghĩa là tôi (I/me)

ANH ĐẦU BẾP DỌN LƯỠI HEO LÊN. ÔNG TA MỚI HỎI NGUYÊN NHÂN TẠI SAO, THÌ ANH ĐẦU BẾP THƯA NGAY RẰNG:"DẠ THƯA ÔNG, KHI NGƯỜI TA THƯỜNG YÊU NHAU, CÁI LƯỠI CỦA HỌ NÓI RA NHỮNG LỜI NGỌT NGÀO NHỨT CHO NHAU. NHƯ VẬY CÁI LƯỠI KHÔNG PHẢI LÀ VẬT NGON NHỨT TRÊN ĐỜI SAO?"

ÔNG PHÚ HỘ CHO CÂU TRẢ LỜI CỦA ANH ĐẦU BẾP THẬT KHÔN NGOAN. VÀI NGÀY SAU ÔNG PHÚ HỘ LẠI GỌI ANH ĐẦU BẾP LÊN VÀ NÓI:"BÂY GIỜ TA MUỐN NẾM MÓN ĂN DỞ NHỨT TRÊN ĐỜI. LÀM ƠN ĐI MUA VỀ NẤU CHO TA".

ANH ĐẦU BẾP VỘI VÀNG RA CHỢ. LẦN NÀY ANH TA KHÔNG PHẢI NGHĨ NGỢI LÂU, ANH ĐI THẲNG ĐẾN HÀNG THỊT VÀ LẠI MUA CÁI LƯỠI HEO LẦN NỮA. ANH ĐEM VỀ NẤU VÀ DỌN LÊN CHO CHỦ ĂN.

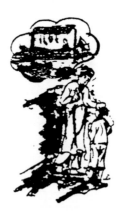

"DẠ THƯA ÔNG, ĐÂY LÀ MÓN DỞ NHÚT TRÊN ĐỜI".

ÔNG PHÚ HỘ LẠI CÀNG NGẠC NHIÊN HƠN KHI TRÔNG THẤY MÓN LƯỠI HEO LẦN NÀY. ÔNG TA MỚI HỎI TẠI SAO LẦN NÀY CÁI LƯỠI LẠI LÀ VẬT DỞ NHÚT TRÊN ĐỜI. ANH TA LIỀN THỦA:

"THƯA ÔNG, KHI NGƯỜI TA GHÉT NHAU, LƯỠI HỌ NÓI RA NHỮNG LỜI XẤU XA NHÚT CHO NHAU. NHƯ VẬY CÁI LƯỠI KHÔNG PHẢI LÀ VẬT DỞ NHÚT TRÊN ĐỜI SAO?"

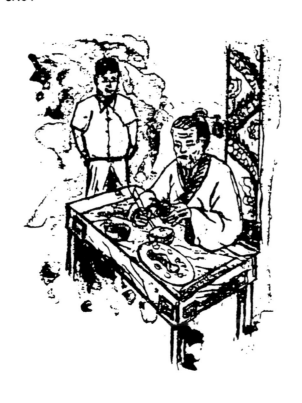

Functional and Nonverbal Assessment

Research in pragmatics has focused on the functions of language and the development of these functions. It has been found that nonverbal communication makes up 65% to 90% of an average message (Katz & Katz, 1983; Knapp, 1978; McCrosky & Wheelers, 1976). Cross-cultural studies on nonverbal communication (Katz & Katz, 1983) reveal that people from different cultures interpret nonverbal signals (e.g., facial expressions) in very different ways, however. The failure to recognize such differences in interpretation may lead to misunderstanding and even communication breakdowns. Clearly, speech-language clinicians must be observant of nonverbal behaviors.

In studying the development of children's language functions, Halliday (1978) found that the first phase occurs between the ages of 10 and 18 months, and involves six functions:

1. instrumental: the language used to satisfy material needs and desires
2. regulatory: the language used to control the behavior of other people
3. interactional: the language used to establish interaction with other people
4. personal: language used for the expression of feelings, attitudes, and interest
5. heuristic: the language used to explore and organize the environment
6. imaginative: the language used to create an imaginary environment

As children grow older, they move into the second phase of development, which generally extends from ages 18 to 36 months. Their language acquires three new functions:

1. pragmatic: the language used to act on the environment. It is a combination of the earlier instrumental, regulatory, and interactional functions.
2. mathetic: the language used to learn about the environment. It grows out of the personal, heuristic, and interactional functions. It is used for such purposes as commenting and recalling.
3. informative: the language used to provide others with new information. This function is represented in references to events that are remote in time or space.

As children pass the age of 3 years, additional language functions can be identified:

1. ideational: the language used to talk about the world, objects, and events. This function grows out of the mathetic function, and it is the representational, cognitive function of language.
2. interpersonal: the language used to participate in the world, communicating with others. It grows out of the earlier pragmatic function, and it is used for social interaction.
3. textual: the language used to express meaning through verbal symbols. This is a function for the expressive use of meaning.

Halliday's (1975) functional model can be used to establish a framework for observing children, specifically, for analyzing their use of language for different communicative intents. Chapman (1981) noted that the communicative intent of 2- to 5-year-olds begins to reflect not only the basic intent of fulfilling their needs, but also a much broader intent of participating in social discourse. The following communicative strategies are used by children in this age group:

1. imitating
2. asking questions
3. expressing needs
4. answering questions
5. describing objects or events
6. describing own acts
7. describing a past experience
8. describing own plan
9. describing a picture book

Checklists based on such a pragmatic model give the clinician, the classroom teacher or aide, and all other informants an opportunity to record their observations and comment on the child's achievement of functional milestones in communication. Checklists may focus on functional communication (Appendix K) or on nonverbal communication (Appendix L). In order to obtain a holistic picture of the child's abilities, however, a teacher or an observer must note a number of basic behaviors:

1. What are the strengths of the child?
2. What are the weaknesses of the child?
3. What are some of the strategies that the child uses to compensate for his weaknesses?
4. What are the discrepancies in different functions of language?
5. What is the attention and concentration level of the child?
6. What methods does the child use to relate to other people?
7. Is the child cooperative?
8. How much confidence does the child have? Does the child need a great deal of encouragement?
9. Does the child need a great deal of structuring?
10. What is the motivational level of the child?
11. How flexible is the child?
12. Is the child tolerant of frustration and failure?
13. How anxious is the child?
14. What is the child's response time (in seconds)?
15. What is the overall energy level of the child?
16. What is the total affect of the child?

Differences vs. Disorders

In recent years, the focus of assessment has been on the communicative demands of particular contexts. Because the communicative act is context-specific, it is reasonable to assume that the communicative difficulties of children will surface when the communicative demand is higher. Thus, if a child is having problems at school, the assessment should be focused on the communicative demands of the classroom.

Asian language minority children who are unfamiliar with the American way of schooling may encounter difficulties when they first attend school in the United States. These difficulties can be overcome with time—unless they are attributable to a language disorder. Therefore, speech-language clinicians must differentiate communication problems that are due to differences in sociocultural linguistic background from those that are due to language disorders.

Because the communicative demands of individual teachers may vary a great deal, language minority children may experience different degrees of difficulties in the different classrooms (Philips, 1983). Iglesias (1985) asserted that the differences in interactions between teachers and the student are related to the child's cultural background and the communicative demands placed on the child by the teachers. Although there are indeed variations in the communicative demands of teachers, certain academic skills are required to perform effectively in school; language minority students must learn these skills.

Children with language disorders fail to understand their role as communicators and the many functions of language use. They use a limited number of communicative strategies and seem to be inflexible and unresponsive at times. The lack of reciprocity and initiation create a communicative breakdown. These children fail to utilize the appropriate linguistic, paralinguistic, social, and pragmatic rules. In other words, these children fail to utilize language effectively and are restricted in their ranges of communicative competence.

Children who fail as communicators generally do not use a variety of communicative strategies and have distinctive communicative styles that create the breakdowns in communication. Cheng (1983) reported some characteristics of their interactional styles:

1. no response to most questions
2. responses to questions only, not to other stimuli
3. most responses not relevant to questions
4. most responses egocentric in nature
5. utterances largely demands
6. use of very few questions
7. few verbal descriptions to accompany their own acts
8. very few commentaries
9. abrupt or negative answers
10. failure to initiate topics
11. failure to maintain topics
12. frequent topic shifts
13. lack of clarifications and elaborations
14. lack of turn-taking and reciprocity
15. lack of overall intelligibility
16. lack of overall productivity

may appear because of cultural background

It is possible that these characteristics appear in the communication of language minority students because of their cultural background. Hispanic LEP children, for example, may not have been asked to recount a past experience and are not asked to label objects at home (Heath, 1984). Chinese children are not generally encouraged to volunteer information or offer commentaries at home (Wong-Fillmore, 1984). Certainly, further research is indicated to identify any social-cultural-linguistic features of language minority children that contribute to their different styles of learning and communication.

Ethnographic analyses raise questions about the validity of traditional test results and the labels given to language minority children based on those results. More refined qualitative measures are needed to ensure that diagnoses are not based on limited background information and a misunderstanding of the dynamics of social interactions.

Conclusion

By observing the child in a holistic fashion and by using multiple observers, the clinician should be able to determine the strengths and weaknesses in the child's communication and to identify the strategies that the child uses to repair any communication breakdowns. Thus, the clinician should be able to supply a summary of the child's skills that includes information about

- the overall productivity of the child (i.e., utterances)
- the overall intelligibility of the child (i.e., articulation, voice)
- the overall linguistic complexity of the child (i.e., syntax, semantics)
- the overall response patterns of the child (i.e., discourse, pragmatics)
- the overall affect of the child, including level of frustration, anxiety, motivation, cooperation, and self-confidence

In assessing the overall communication of children, the clinician must pay attention to their nonverbal paralinguistic features, kinesics, and proxemics, as well as to their receptive language and expressive language. The clinician also needs to understand their use of metalinguistic features, their pragmatic use of language, and, in general, their use of content.

CHAPTER 10

Intervention Issues and Procedures

It is unrealistic to expect that monolingual English-speaking speech-language pathologists can quickly attain linguistic competence in the Asian languages because (1) there are so many of these languages, (2) they are difficult to learn; and (3) there are only a limited number of programs that offer instruction in such languages. Yet, monolingual English-speaking speech-language pathologists must find ways to provide quality service to Asian language minority children so that they are able to become linguistically and communicatively competent.

Working with Asian Families

Family members can serve as facilitators in providing remediation at home. In order to work with parents, however, speech-language clinicians must take into consideration certain differences in orientation between American and Asian views (Table 10-1). It is important for clinicians to understand that Asian parents generally restrain themselves from expressing their feelings. Even when they are anxious, depressed, angry, hostile, or strongly opposed to the clinician's recommendations, their facial expressions are usually neutral. Most clinicians hope to establish rapport with the parents by using open, two-way communication; however, Asian parents are more comfortable with one-way communication, readily accepting advice and suggestions from school authorities. They are not accustomed to the loosely structured American way of dealing with parents and respond better to more well-defined patterns of interaction. As a result of these cultural features, school personnel sometimes find it difficult to determine whether Asian parents are in agreement with their comments. Like all parents, these parents, are caring and will do everything they can to help their children succeed in school.

Working with Asian Students

It is necessary for Asian language minority students to learn the social, pragmatic, and discourse rules of American schools and for speech-language clinicians to learn the social, cultural, and pragmatic rules of the Asian culture. Because their unfamiliarity with the sociocultural discourse rules of English may result in ineffective

Table 10-1 Working with Parents with Different Views

American View	Asian View
Individual-centered	Family-oriented
Verbal/emotional behavior expressed	Restraint of feelings
Two-way communication	Silence as an indication of respect
	One-way communication from authority
Working together	Advice seeking
Loosely defined patterns of interaction	Well-defined patterns of interaction
Open discussion	Private vs. public display of shame/pride/disgrace—shame, pride, and disgrace are not displayed publicly.
Clear distinctions between physical and mental well-being	Physical and mental well-being are defined differently—only physical illness is considered a sickness.
Active involvement of parents	Appearance of passivity and uninvolvement

communication, Asian students should be trained explicitly in these rules. Intervention strategies should be geared toward the cultural/social and ecological environment of the school and the classroom. In order to intervene effectively, speech-language clinicians should become sensitive to cultural differences.

Teacher observations of the overt classroom behaviors of Asian students can be misinterpreted, causing further miscommunication and conflict (Table 10-2). Teachers and others who work with the Asian child need to be aware of these

Table 10-2 Misinterpretations of Overt Classroom Behaviors

Observed Behavior	Teacher's Perception
Child is quiet.	Child is passive.
Child keeps distance.	Child is afraid of him or her.
Child speaks only when asked a question.	Child is not interested.
Child will not make a choice.	Child is defiant.
Child looks down when scolded.	Child is defiant.
Child does not look at the teacher.	Child has poor eye contact.
Child observes and does not participate in activities.	Child is shy and inhibited.
Child does not ask questions or volunteer information.	Child lacks initiative.
Child sits by himself or herself.	Child does not participate in activities.
Child does not defend himself or herself.	Child is a pushover.
Child is alone.	Child has difficulty making friends.
Child waits for teacher's directions rather than making a choice.	Child is indecisive.
Child observes and imitates.	Child lacks creativity.
Child does not know what to do when not told exactly what to do.	Child is dependent on adults.
Child does not talk back.	Child is submissive.
Child does not have many friends.	Child is shy and not sociable.
Child cries and is withdrawn.	Child is undisciplined.
Child hits other children.	Child is aggressive.
Child accepts unwelcome activities.	Child does not say what he or she wants to do.
Child asks a mediator to approach the adult, instead of confronting the adult directly.	Child will not seek help.
Child is courteous to authority and not assertive.	Child needs to learn to be assertive and initiate.

possible misperceptions and to be sensitive to the child's need to be accepted as a student at the school. Asian language minority children are often caught in cultural conflicts, and educators should assist them and guide them through the difficult process of acculturation.

The following guidelines will help to prepare speech-language clinicians to work with the Asian language minority child in the classroom:

1. Show the child respect as an individual with a unique background by
   - approaching the child as an individual, getting to know his or her individual needs and family. Overt concern is evidence of a personal relationship, and making the relationship personalized is very important to the Asian person.
   - making an effort to meet the child's parents and, if possible, paying a home visit
   - setting up a buddy system to make the child feel a part of the school and to provide more opportunities for the child to make friends
   - incorporating aspects of different cultures into lesson plans to encourage understanding of cultural diversity
   - encouraging the child to show talents in class, thereby improving the child's self-image and increasing his or her status in the class
2. Be cautious with words, taking care to avoid speaking too frankly.
3. Reprimand the child for physical aggression in private, explaining the behaviors and rules that are acceptable to class members.
4. Reinforce verbally the child's willingness to cooperate and share in order to enhance the child's self-esteem.
5. Try to arrange seating so that the child will be seated near children who are less aggressive and tend to be more helpful to make the child feel comfortable and less shy.
6. Provide the child with opportunities to make simple decisions and choices, show approval of the child's decisions, and guide the child from making simple to more complex decisions.
7. Tell the child what makes a good student.
8. Allow the child to function in a group to gain confidence.
9. Recognize the child's use of an intermediary as his or her way of asking for attention; explain privately that he or she should feel free to approach the teacher at any time.*

Working with Multiple Informants

Although unable to speak the language of the Asian language minority client, the clinician is trained in language development and language disorders. Thus, with the assistance of bilingual teachers and aides, as well as children in the school who speak the mother tongue of the child in question, the clinician can provide remediation to the Asian children. In addition, family members can be used to facilitate assessment, remediation, and communication. In other words, the speech-language pathologist is not the primary provider of remediation, but rather the secondary provider of remediation. Those individuals who speak the

---

*Parts of the content were taken from the cultural materials of ICP, San Diego State University.

native language of the child become the facilitators, the interactants, the partners, and the informants.

The multiple partners/multiple informant approach is extremely useful for the many speech-language pathologists who work in isolated areas and do not have bilingual resources and personnel support in the school system. The various informants serve various functions, depending on their level of training and expertise (Table 10-3).

The speech pathologist can remediate some disorders by working as a consultant to the bilingual teaching staff, who actually provide the language model for the child. When a child has an articulation problem, for example, it is advisable to use a bilingual teacher, a bilingual aide, or a bilingual resource teacher as the primary provider for remediation.

A 7-year-old Vietnamese boy was referred for speech therapy because his speech was largely unintelligible. His resource teacher, a Vietnamese, served as an informant, interpreter, and facilitator throughout the diagnostic and information-gathering session. By comparing a speech sample of the child to a speech sample of the resource teacher and with the help of the resource teacher, the speech clinician was able to pinpoint the child's articulation problem—an inability to produce the liquid phoneme l and the retroflex phoneme r. The child substituted w for the r and l phonemes. Through the bilingual resource teacher, the speech clinician was able to demonstrate the place and manner of articulation of the two phonemes in question. By means of oral motor drills and drills on the phonemes, the child learned correct production of the r and the l phonemes in Vietnamese. Although the initial r phoneme in Vietnamese is qualitatively different from the English r phoneme, the establishment of the retroflex sound in Vietnamese was very helpful to the child in later establishing the correct production of the r phoneme in English.

Thus, the first part of therapy was conducted in Vietnamese through the translation of the bilingual resource teacher, the second part of therapy was devoted to the production of the targeted English phoneme. The Vietnamese resource teacher served as a resource person throughout the course of therapy. In this case, the speech-language pathologist played two roles: (1) the role of a diagnostician and therapist, and (2) the role of consultant. By utilizing the language expertise of the resource teacher, the clinician was successful in providing therapy to the child.

Table 10-3 Possible Functions of Multiple Informants

Informant	Function
Older sibling	Provide language modeling and comment on the child's language
Parents	Comment on the child's language at home and in comparison to that of siblings
Monolingual peers	Comment on interaction
Monolingual teachers	Comment on overall behavior, academic skills, learning style, learning attention
Bilingual upper grade schoolmate	Comment on native language fluency and provide articulation and language model
Bilingual teacher (aide)	Comment on native language acquisition and competency, conduct assessment and remediation
Bilingual psychologist	Provide psychological profile
Linguist	Comment on features of native language
ESL teacher	Comment on acquisition of English compared to other children
Foreign students	Comment on native language of the student

The discourse framework developed by Heath (1985) indicates that children are expected to use language for several common purposes:

1. to label and describe objects, events, and information
2. to recap or recast past events in a predictable order and format
3. to follow directions for oral and written activities without sustained personal reinforcement from adults and peers
4. to sustain and maintain social interactions of the group
5. to obtain information from nonintimates
6. to account for unique experiences, to link these experiences to generally known ideas or events, and even to create new information or to indicate ideas in innovative ways

Using Heath's model, the speech-language clinician can adopt, adapt, and create strategies for eliciting the different types of discourse patterns:

1. label guests. The child may be given the names of items or asked the names of items. For example, Who's that? What's that? What color is it?
2. meaning quests. The meaning of the child's utterance is inferred. For example, a mother may say, "Open? You want to open the box?" In school, teachers do the same, asking students to explain the meaning of words, pictures, etc.
3. recounts. The speaker retells experiences or discusses information known to both himself and the listener. The child displays knowledge through oral or written work.
4. accounts. The speaker provides information that is new to the listener. For example, activities such as "show and tell" are considered accounting.
5. eventcasts. The speaker provides a narrative of an event currently in the attention of both himself and the listener. This narrative may be simultaneous with the event or before the event. For example, children may talk about what is happening as they play with toys. Adults may talk about the steps required in an event, such as preparing certain foods.
6. story-telling. Stories written in the child's own language can be used to further their knowledge base and communication skills. Parents, teachers, teacher's aides, or siblings or peers may ask the child to talk about a story, to retell the story, or to fill in blanks or answer questions about the story. Because this activity is familiar in all Asian cultures, everyone can help. As long as language stimulation and modeling is sufficient, the monolingual speech-language pathologist can serve as a consultant and an occasional interactant, rather than an interventionist.

Since all these activities are best carried out in the context of the classroom, it is essential for the monolingual speech-language pathologist to work with the classroom teachers and aides to provide them with ideas, materials, and strategies to elicit responses from the children who are in need of language services.

The purpose of a remediation program is to increase the intelligibility and productivity of the individual child, and to increase the quality and quantity of communication. Thus, language remediation should provide the child with ample opportunities to interact and use language as a social tool. Because discourse is the basis for interaction, it is wise to concentrate on discourse strategies to help a child overcome speech and language problems.

General Strategies

In any remediation program, it is essential to create a communication-rich, as well as a cognitively demanding, environment. Exposing children to different situations and arranging for them to have different partners can modify their behaviors. For example, very quiet children may become quite talkative, even volunteering information. It is important to structure scenes to stimulate the interest of the children, such as asking them to role-play, to give instructions, or to solve problems.

Asian children need direct encouragement to participate in communicative acts. They function better when the clinician is able to provide contexts that are comfortable and familiar to them, at the same time providing challenging and novel experiences. Each child must be motivated to talk and to feel good about himself or herself, to feel that it is good to talk and communicate effectively. The encouragement of parents, teachers, siblings, and others plays a significant role in a child's successful communication.

The clinician should be sensitive to children's need to create their own meaning based on their own frames of reference. The testing environment and learning environment should be adjusted to accommodate each child's individual needs. For example, a child may bring a pair of chopsticks to a session and show the clinician how to use them. If the clinician is unable to pick up food by using the chopsticks, the child has an opportunity to teach the clinician how to use them.

Language proficiency must be learned through practice. It is imperative that Asian language minority children have ample opportunities to practice and use the language. Nursery rhymes are excellent ways of practicing the language, and words that rhyme are also ideal in arousing children's curiosity and interest. Some children do not participate in games, group activities, and stories because they are unfamiliar. It is useful to play games, especially those that require planning and manipulation of objects, and those that are a little difficult. Some suggested ideas for activities are:

- work on a multicultural calendar
- use cooperative learning strategies
- work on collective story building
- adopt an experiential approach
- use personal life history
- use personal weather report (showing personal feelings)
- let the children lead the way
- let the children choose their activity (story, game, play, etc.)
- bring multiculturalism into the classroom

Interesting toys should be an integral part of remediation. Children need to play and explore the world. Toys such as Lego blocks, puzzles, toys that make noise, toys that have detachable parts, toys that move, toys that are identical, toys that are almost identical, toys that have missing parts, and toys that have broken parts may stimulate conversation. Books and personal photographs may be useful. Clay, crayons, and paints should be available for children to create pictures and objects, and to make stories. A sand box can also be useful. Reading and writing instructions can be embedded in a meaningful context based on the child's previous experiences.

The clinician should read to the child and introduce new vocabulary in context, acting out verbs and using them in multiple contexts. Halliday (1963) suggested that clinicians capitalize on a child's imagination to create situations and activities conducive for the use of language.

In summary, intervention procedures for Asian students of limited English proficiency should be based on the clinician's knowledge of their linguistic, cognitive, and sociocultural background. Monolingual speech-language clinicians need to nurture their own growth in cross-cultural communicative competence in order to help these children resolve their conflicts and confusions.

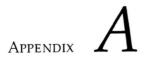

Assessment Procedures

	Done	More work needed	Further assessment
1. *Information Gathering* Medical Information			
Child questionnaire (*See Appendix D.*)			
School records Present Past			
ESL information			
2. *Consultation/conference* Teacher(s)			
Resource teacher			
ESL teacher			
Parents (*See Appendix C.*)			
Other school personnel Speech pathologist Psychologist Social worker Native speaker (child's L1)			
Others (sibling, friends, etc.)			
3. *Systematic Observation* Classroom Teacher-child Child-other children			
ESL classroom Teacher-child Child-other children			
Playground			
Home Parent-child Child-sibling Child-others			

(continued)

	Done	More work needed	Further assessment
4. *Assessment of Communicative Abilities*			
English speech-language testing			
Receptive vocabulary			
Syntax			
Articulation			
Auditory comprehension			
Narration			
Pragmatics			
Expressive vocabulary			
Language sample			
Speech-language testing in L_2			
Articulation			
Syntax			
Auditory comprehension			
Cloze procedure			
Cognitive-functional			
Nonverbal communication			
Language sample			
Oral-peripheral			
Hearing screening			
Vision screening			
Educational testing in L_1			
Psychological testing			
Reading			
Writing			
Mathematics			
Other			

Adult Questionnaire

Name: _____ Sex:_____
       Family   Given   Middle

Address: _____ Telephone: _____
_____ Ethnicity: _____

Date of Birth: _____ Age: _____ Place of birth: _____
Country of origin: _____
Names of parents: Father: _____ Ethnicity: _____
                  Mother: _____ Ethnicity: _____
Are you married? Yes _____ No _____ If yes, how long have you been
married? _____
Name of spouse: _____ Age: _____
Education level of spouse: _____ Occupation: _____
Do you have children? Yes _____ No _____ If yes, how many? _____
Names of children: _____ Age: _____
                         _____ Age: _____
                         _____ Age: _____
                         _____ Age: _____
                         _____ Age: _____

What language(s) do you speak? _____
What language is spoken at home? _____
Did you learn any English before you came? Yes _____ No _____
If yes, where did you learn it? _____ How long? _____
How old were you when you learned English? _____
Who taught you English? _____
How were you taught? _____
_____

How do you rate your English proficiency? _____

	Excellent	Good	Fair	Poor
Reading	_____	_____	___	___
Speaking	_____	_____	___	___
Writing	_____	_____	___	___
Comprehension	_____	_____	___	___

If you know little or no English, who does the talking for you? _____

Time of arrival in the U.S.A.: _____ Age: _____
How long have you been here? _____ years _____ months
When did you leave your place of origin? _____
Why did you come to the U.S.A.? _____

Are you an immigrant? Yes _____ No _____
Refugee? Yes _____ No _____
What is your level of education? _____
What is your occupation? _____
Is English required at your work setting? Yes _____ No _____
If yes, how much English is required? _____
Did you take English classes after you came to the U.S.A.?
Yes _____ No _____
If yes, how long? _____ With whom? _____
How much English is required for your everyday activity? _____

Background Information Questionnaire

Instructions: We are going to ask you some questions about your child's medical history, educational history, and related areas. Please be as thorough as you can in your remarks. If I am not clear, please stop me and ask me to say it again. If you don't feel comfortable in answering the question, please let me know. All we want to do here is to obtain as much background information as possible, and, since you are the child's parent, we feel that you have much to contribute.

1. When was your child born? _____
2. Was this a hospital? _____
3. How was the pregnancy? _____
   How was your health during pregnancy? _____
   _____
4. How was the delivery? _____
5. Were any instruments used? _____
6. Were there any postnatal complications? _____
7. How was your child's physical development? _____
   _____
   Were there any handicapping conditions? _____
   If yes, who made the diagnosis? _____
   When? _____ How did you feel about it? _____
   _____
8. Was your child ever hospitalized? _____ If yes, where? _____
   When? _____ Why? _____ How long? _____
   Who was the physician? _____
9. Were there problems in feeding? _____
10. Were there any prolonged illnesses? _____
    High fever? _____ Accidents? _____
11. Has his/her hearing been checked? _____
12. Has his/her vision been checked? _____
13. Has he/she seen a dentist? _____
    What is the condition of his/her teeth? _____
14. What is his/her diet history? _____
    _____

15. How is his/her diet now? _____
16. Does he/she have a pediatrician? _____
    Who? _____
    Has your child seen any other medical specialist? _____
    If yes, Who? _____
    When? _____ Where? _____ Why? _____
17. When did you come to the United States? _____
    Why did you come? _____
    For refugees: Was he/she ever in a refugee camp? _____
    How long? _____ Tell us about it. _____
    _____
    _____
18. Was he/she ever on a boat? _____ How long? _____
    Tell us about it. _____
    _____
19. How many brothers and sisters does he/she have? _____
    Are they all here? _____
20. Are there any family members who had or have difficulty in speaking or hear-
    ing, or problems such as mental retardation, cerebral palsy, cleft palate, or
    stuttering? _____
    If yes, please explain. _____
    _____
21. Was your child ever in school? _____ Where? _____ How long? _____
22. How was his/her performance in school? _____
    Grade? _____
23. Do you have a report from the school? _____ Any comments from the
    teacher? _____
24. Was he/she involved in special programs? _____
    How did he/she do? _____
25. Was he/she in a day-care or child care program? _____
    If yes, how did he/she do? _____
26. Did he/she repeat a grade? _____ If yes, why? _____
    _____
27. How was the program similar to his/her program now? _____
    How was the program different from his/her program now? _____
28. How many are living in your home? _____
29. Who takes care of your child after school? _____
30. Who makes the decisions at home? _____
31. Does your child have his/her own room? _____
    If no, who does your child share the room with? _____ Where does
    he/she study? _____
32. Does your child mostly play inside the house? _____ Outside? _____ By
    himself/herself? _____ With a sibling? _____
33. Who does he/she play with? _____
    Are they older or younger? _____
    How does he/she play? _____
34. What does he/she like to play? _____
    What toys do you have? _____
    Does he/she read? _____ What books and magazines do you have? _____
35. Do you work? _____ If yes, what do you do? _____

When are you home? _____

36. Does your spouse work? _____ If yes, what does he/she do? _____ When is he/she home? _____
37. What is your educational background? _____
    Your spouse's educational background? _____
38. What language(s) is used at home? _____
39. When did your child say his/her first word? _____
    How do you feel about his/her speech now? _____
    _____
40. Do you feel that your child understands everything you say? _____
    Explain. _____
    _____
41. What language does he/she speak when he/she responds to you? _____
42. Does your child speak your native language with his siblings? _____
    Friends? _____
43. Do your children speak your native language or English among themselves?
    _____
44. Do you help your child with homework? _____
45. How do you feel about his/her maintenance of your native language? _____
    Do you send him/her to language school during the weekend? _____
46. What do you expect the school to do for your child? _____
47. Do you attend any social function? _____ Where? _____
    With whom? _____ What are your leisure activities? _____
48. Do you have difficulty disciplining your child? _____ His/her siblings? _____
49. What responsibilities are placed on your child? _____
    _____
    On his/her siblings? _____
50. Does he/she dress himself? _____
51. Does he/she know your telephone number and address? _____
52. Do you read to him/her? _____ What are his/her favorite stories? _____
    Can he/she tell the story back to you? _____
53. Does he/she watch TV? _____ What is his/her favorite program? _____
54. Do you think your child is a hard worker? _____
    If so, why? _____
    Do you think your child is lazy? _____ Why? _____
    _____

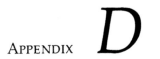
Child Questionnaire

Name: _____ Sex: _____
       Family   Given   Middle

Address: _____Telephone: _____
_____ Ethnicity: _____
Date of birth: _____ Age: _____ Place of birth: _____
Country of origin: _____
Names of parents: Father: _____ Age: _____ Ethnicity: _____
   Education level: _____ Occupation: _____
           Mother: _____ Age: _____ Ethnicity: _____
   Education level: _____ Occupation: _____
Do you have siblings? Yes _____ No _____ If yes, how many: _____
Names of siblings:
_____ Age: _____ Education level: _____
_____ Age: _____ Education level: _____
_____ Age: _____ Education level: _____
_____ Age: _____ Education level: _____
_____ Age: _____ Education level: _____
What languages do the siblings speak to the child? _____

_____ _____ _____ _____
Language(s) spoken at home: _____
Did the child learn any English before he/she came? Yes _____ No _____
If yes, when did he/she learn it? _____ For how long? _____
Time of arrival in the U.S.A.: _____ Age: _____
How long has the child been here? _____years _____months
Why did the child come to the U.S.A.? _____
Immigration? _____ Refugee? _____
For refugees only: Was the child in a camp? Yes _____ No _____
If yes, where was the camp? _____
How long was he/she in the camp? _____
Who sponsored him/her to come to the U.S.A.? _____

How did the child get to the camp? _____
Describe briefly his/her experiences at the camp. _____

_____
_____

Cognitive-Ecological-Functional Questionnaire

Objects needed: 5 crayons (red, yellow, blue, black, white), 1 long, 1 broken, 1 bigger; a picture with just a face; a picture of body parts; a blank piece of paper; 2 cups, one with some water; clay.

Questions for the Child

1. What's your name? _____
   Do you have an English name? _____
2. How old are you? _____
3. When is your birthday? _____
   What grade are you in? _____ What is the name of your teacher? _____
4. Where do you live? _____
5. Do you know your telephone number? _____
   What is it? _____
6. Do you have brothers and sisters? _____ Tell me about them. _____
   _____
7. Who do you live with? _____
8. What does your daddy do? _____
9. What does your mommy do? _____
10. Do you have friends? _____
11. What are their names? _____
12. What is your favorite toy? _____ Tell me about it. _____
13. What is your favorite game? _____
    Tell me how you play that game. _____
    _____
14. What is your favorite food? _____
15. What is your favorite TV show? _____
    Tell me about it. _____
    _____
16. What is your favorite story? _____
    Tell me about it. _____
    _____
17. What is your favorite book? _____

Tell me about it. _____

18. (*Produce crayons.*) Which one is bigger? _____
19. Which one is broken? _____ Which one is longer? _____
20. Which one is red? _____ yellow? _____ blue? _____
    black? _____ white? _____
21. Give me two? _____ three? _____ five? _____ one? _____
    five? _____ Make 2 groups, 1 and 4.
    Which one has more? _____
22. What are they for? _____
23. (*Produce paper.*) Draw a house for me.
24. Draw a man for me.
25. (*Produce picture of a face.*) Look at this picture. What is missing? _____
    Can you draw the parts on? _____
26. (*Produce picture of a person.*) Can you name the parts of the body?
    _____
27. Show me your left hand _____ right hand _____
28. (*Produce cups.*) What is this for? _____ What is in this cup? _____
29. Pour the water from one cup to the other. Which one has more water? _____
30. Put the crayons in front of the paper _____ on top of the paper _____
    under the paper _____ in the cup _____ beside the paper _____
31. (*Produce clay.*) I am going to make a ball. Can you make a ball? _____ I am
    going to make a snake. Can you make a snake? _____ Tell me how you can
    make a snake. _____

Assessment of Communicative Abilities

Linguistic

	Done	Need More Assessment
I. Receptive		
A. Oral		
1. vocabulary		
2. syntax		
3. narrative		
B. Written		
1. vocabulary		
2. syntax		
3. narrative		
4. spelling		
II. Expressive		
A. Oral		
1. vocabulary		
2. syntax		
3. pragmatics		
a. communicative functions		
i. accounting		
ii. recounting		
iii. label quest		
iv. meaning quest		
v. eventcasting		
vi. story-telling		
b. discourse skills		
i. attention		
ii. turn allocation		
iii. topic coherence		

	Done	Need More Assessment
iv. repair		
v. role adjustment		
vi. topic initiation		
v. topic maintenance		
c. metalinguistic skills		
i. comment about language		
ii. language games		
iii. word play		
iv. identification of sounds, words, parts of speech		

Nonlinguistic

	Done	Need More Assessment
I. Nonverbal communication		
A. Paralanguage		
1. pitch		
2. stress		
3. intonation		
4. vocal		
B. Kinesics		
1. gesture		
2. body movement		
3. facial expressions		
4. gazing		
5. posture		
C. Proxemics		
1. use of personal and social space		
2. level of comfort		
D. Overall affect		

Assessment of Overall Behavioral Pattern

Name: _____

Date of birth: _____ Today's date: _____

Observer: _____

Informant: _____

Relationship: _____ Native Language: _____

	Yes	No
1. Frequently chooses to play alone	—	—
2. Frequently uses gestures or other nonverbal communication, interrupting speech	—	—
3. Frequently speaks in single words or short phrases	—	—
4. Frequently chooses to sit in areas away from the main activity, such as in the corner or in the back of the room	—	—
5. Frequently remains silent during sharing time	—	—
6. Frequently fails to follow instructions and directions	—	—
7. Frequently speaks in telegraphic speech (e.g., omits words, parts of words)	—	—
8. Frequently mixes up sounds in words	—	—
9. Frequently misunderstands words	—	—
10. Has difficulty remembering words, things, and events	—	—
11. Uses immature or improper words	—	—
12. Frequently gives improper responses	—	—
13. Frequently stutters or stammers	—	—
14. Speaks in a way that is difficult to understand	—	—
15. Speaks in an extremely loud voice	—	—
16. Complains of earaches	—	—
17. Holds head in a particular position when spoken to	—	—
18. Watches speaker's face closely when spoken to	—	—
19. Appears to be hearing some things and not others	—	—
20. Has a voice that is raspy, breathy, hoarse, etc.	—	—

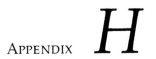

Articulation Tests

Articulation Test: Vietnamese

				RESPONSE		
Sounds: CONSONANTS				ISO	WD	COMMENTS
IPA	SPEL	KEY-WORD	MEANING			
p	p	ép	to force			
b	b	ba	three			
t	t	to	big			
t'	th	thu	autumn			
ʈ	tr	tre	bamboo			not in Northern dialects; replaced by /c/
d	đ	đu	swing			
c	ch	cha	father			
k	c,k	ca	sing			
kp̂	c	học	study			
g	g,gh	gan	liver			
m	m	ma	ghost			
n	n	nó	he/she			
ɲ	nh	nhà	house			
ŋ	ng ngh	nga	swan			
ŋm	ng	lông	hair			
f	ph	phá	destroy			
v	v	voi	elephant			not in Southern dialect; replaced by /j/
s	x	xa	far			
z	d,gi	dê già	goat old			only in the Northern dialect; replaced by /j/ in Central and Southern dialects
ʃ	s	sao	star			not in Northern dialect

(continued)

Articulation Test: Vietnamese continued

				RESPONSE		
Sounds: CONSONANTS				ISO	WD	COMMENTS
IPA	SPEL	KEY-WORD	MEANING			
ʒ	r	ruồi	flies			in Central and Southern dialects only
j	d,gi	dê	goat			in Central and Southern dialects only
x	kh	khi	monkey			
l	l	lá	leaf			
r	r	ruồi	flies			in some dialects, not a regular phoneme
w	o,u	hoa	flower			
y	i	tai	ear			

Source: Used with permission of Huynh Dinh Te.

				RESPONSE		
Sounds: VOWELS				ISO	WD	COMMENTS
IPA	SPEL	KEY-WORD	MEANING			
i	i	đi	go			
e	ê	lê	pear			
ɛ	e	nghe	hear			
a	a	ma	ghost			
u	u	thu	autumn			
o	ô	khô	dry			
ɔ	o	to	big			
ɯ	u	thu	mail			
ɤ	o	mo	dream			
ʌ	â	sân	yard			
ɐ	ă	bắp	corn			

				RESPONSE		
Sound: Stimulus Word				ISO	WD	COMMENTS
CPA	Pinyin	Chinese	English			
ㄅ	b	ba 爸爸 bà	father			
ㄆ	p	pó 婆婆 pò	grand-mother			
ㄉ	d	dì 弟弟 di	younger-brother			
ㄊ	t	tài 太太 tai	wife			
ㄍ	g	gē 哥哥 gè	older-brother			
ㄎ	k	kē 可可 kè	but			
ㄐ	j	jiě 姊姊 jiè	older-sister			
ㄑ	q	qīn 親親 qin	kiss			
ㄒ	x	xìe 謝謝 xie	thanks			
ㄗ	z	zǒu 走走 zóu	walk			
ㄘ	c	cǎo 草草 cáo	grass			
ㄙ	s	saǒ 嫂嫂 saó	sister-in-law			
ㄓ	zh	zhǎo 找著 zhe	find			
ㄔ	ch	chǎng 常常 chǎng	often			
ㄕ	sh	shū 叔叔 shú	uncle			
ㄖ	r	rén 人人 rén	people			
ㄇ	m	mǎi 買賣 mài	business			
ㄋ	n	níu 牛奶 naí	milk			
ㄌ	l	lì 力量 liàng	power			
ㄈ	h	fáng 方法 fǎ	method			
ㄈ	f	hén 很好 hǎo	very-good			

Sample Pictures To Be Used for Language Elicitation

The pictures in this Appendix can be used in assessment with children from Asian language backgrounds. Objects, activities, and symbols are shown that have relevance to the cultural experiences of Asian children. These pictures may be reproduced for use in assessmemt. Brief descriptions of each picture are presented below:

> *Picture 1*- In this picture, the people are celebrating the Chinese New Year.

> *Picture 2*- In this picture, symbols of luck are presented for the Chinese New Year Celebration.

> *Picture 3*- In this picture, the lion dancers are performing the traditional lion dance.

> *Picture 4*- In this picture, the mother is serving traditional "Northern style" Chinese noodles and dumplings.

> *Picture 5*- In this picture, the mother is serving steamed rice, fish, and vegetables for dinner.

> *Picture 6*- In this picture, the lady is playing a traditional Lao musical instrument.

> *Picture 7*- In this picture, a mother and her child are paying respect to the Buddha.

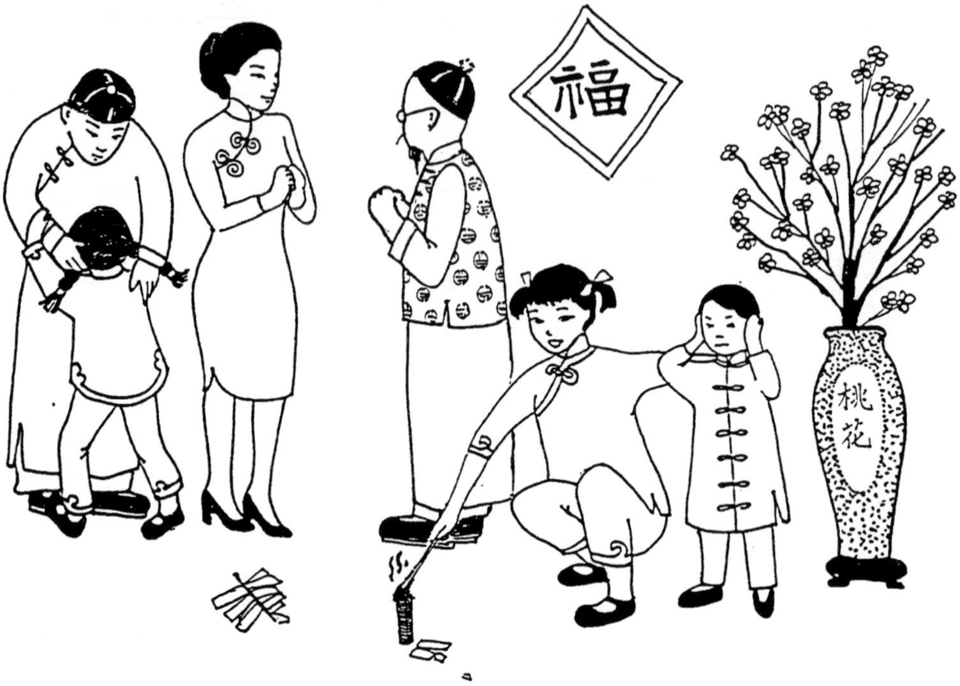
福
桃花

Picture 1

____

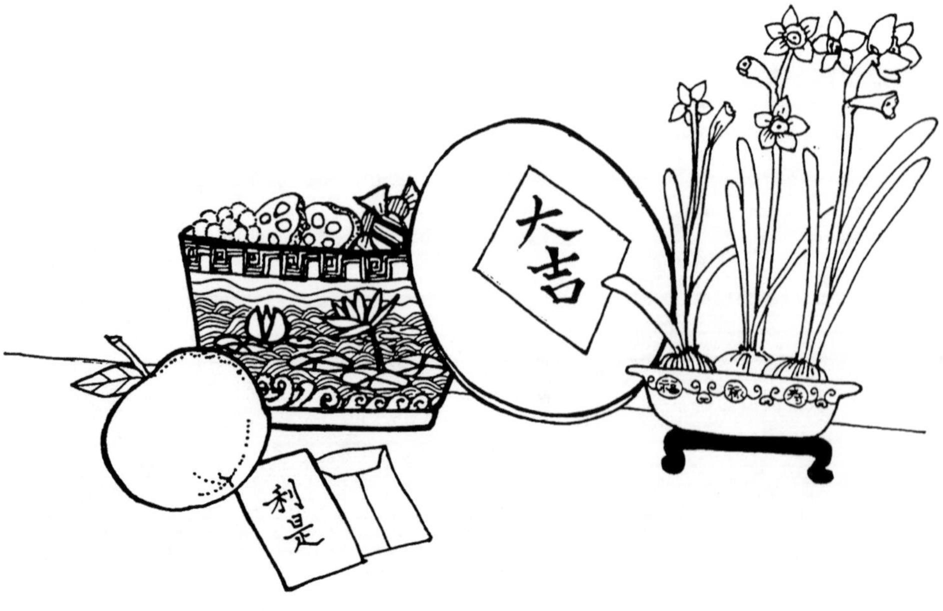
大吉
利是

Picture 2

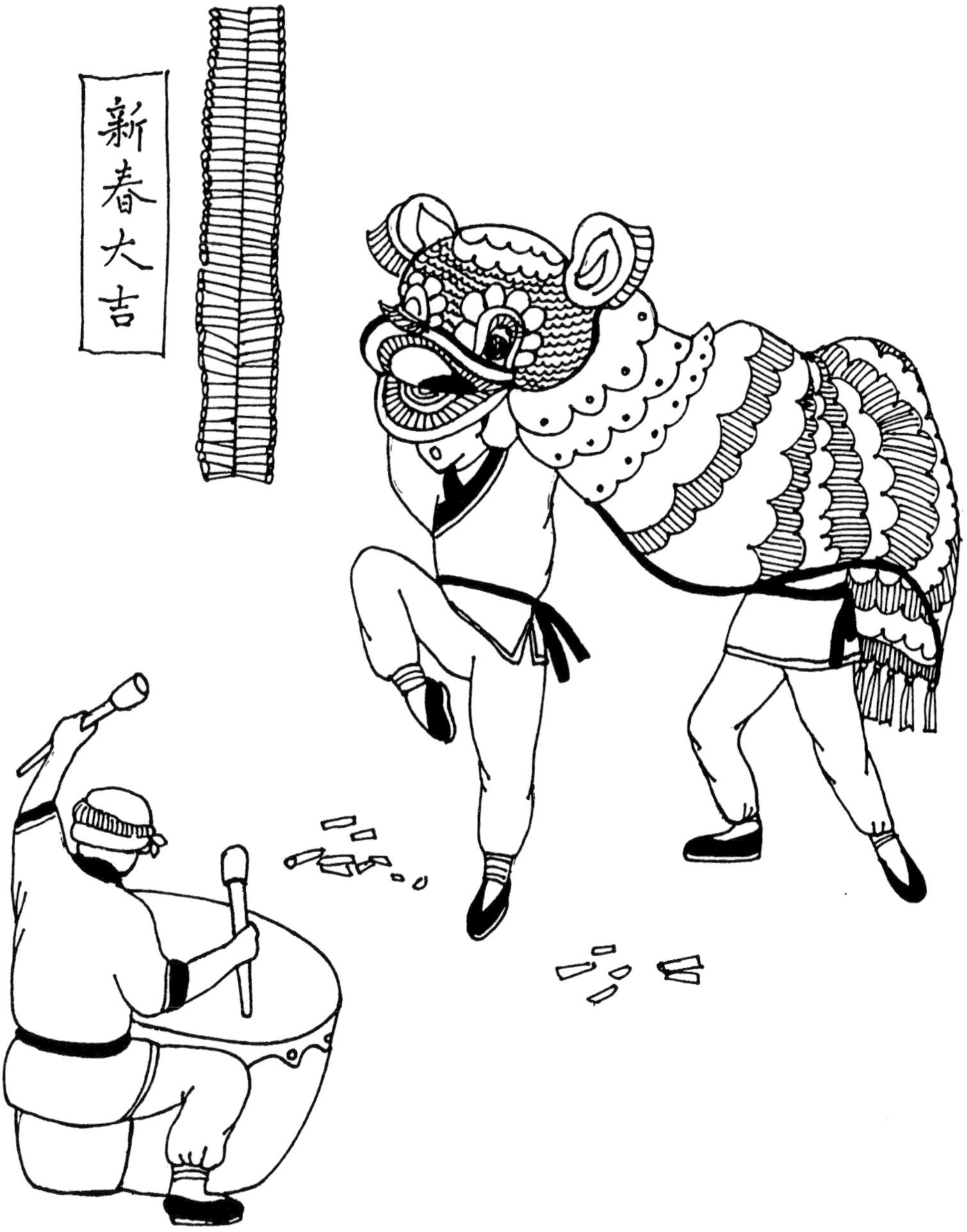
新春大吉

Picture 3

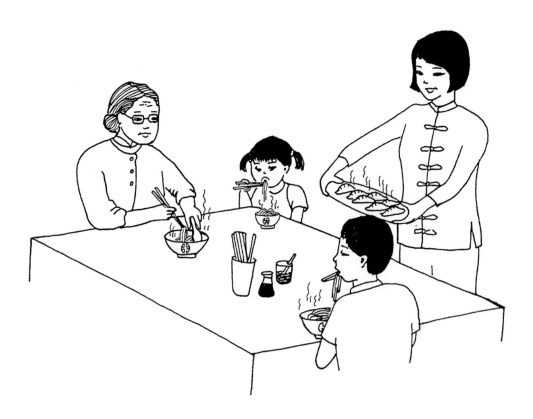

Picture 4

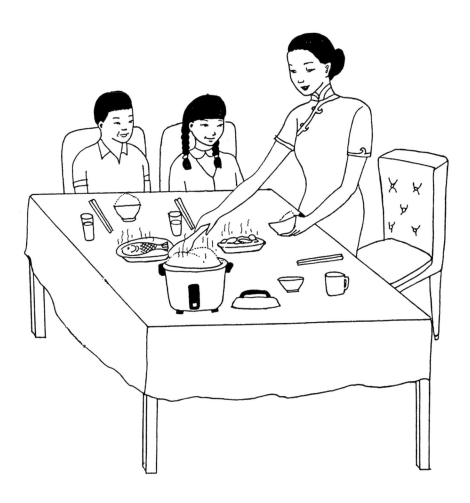

Picture 5

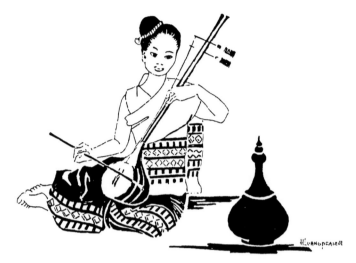

ວິ ຊຸ

Picture 6

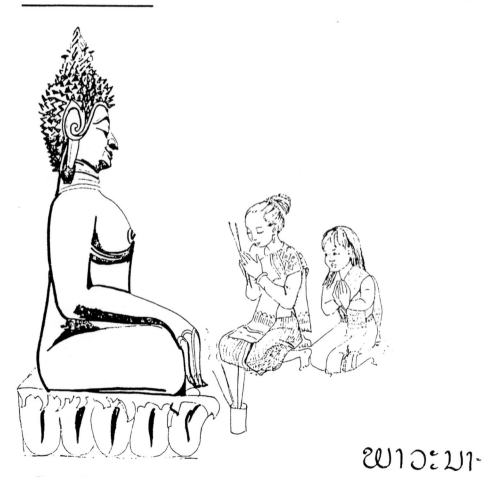

ພາວະນາ

Picture 7

Sample Stories for Language Assessment

When using short stories in language assessment, it is important to examine the appropriateness of the story content and to make changes in the content to reflect the experiences of the children being tested. Examples of short stories are presented in this Appendix.

Story 1

The children liked their teacher. She was such a good teacher. Each child wanted to give her a present. Rich brought her some cheese. Carol chose some peaches. Charlie gave the teacher an egg. Why did Charlie choose an egg? All the children laughed at Charlie. The teacher wouldn't like such a present. The teacher sat down in her chair. The teacher watched the egg. The teacher and the children saw the egg move. Suddenly, the egg hatched a chicken. The teacher saw the baby chick. The teacher loved Charlie's present.

Questions that may be asked include the following:

Who wanted to give the teacher a present?
Who brought the egg?
Who laughed at Charlie?
Who saw the egg move?
What did the teacher see?

The pictures on the following pages show an adaptation of this story for Chinese students. In the original story, one boy gave the teacher a piece of cheese. In the Chinese version, the cheese was changed to peaches because peaches are a traditional birthday symbol. Cheese is not used in China.

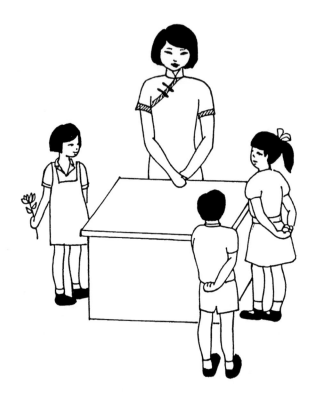

老師今天過生日, 方大才
帶了一個鶏蛋給她, 張竹敏
帶了一朵花給她, 馬思琦
帶了兩個桃子給她.

忽然間, 那個蛋開始動了.
動得很快.

一下子, 蛋殻裂開了, 一支
小鶏跑出來了, 老師看了,
很高興, 就把小鶏抱在手中.

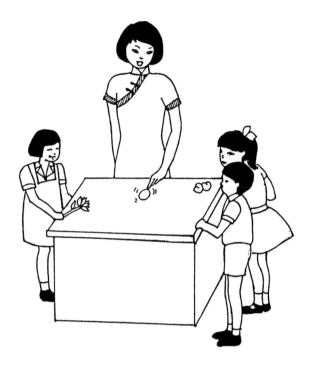

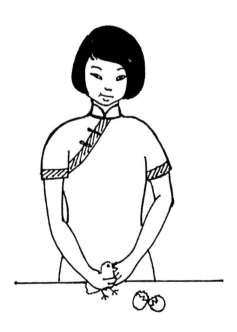

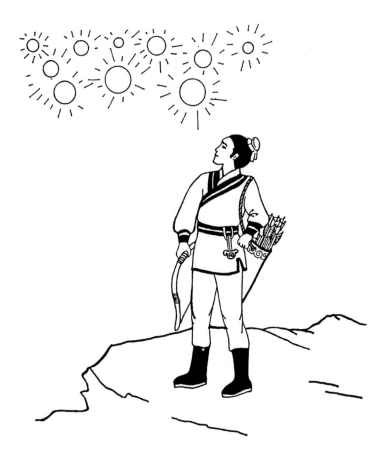

Story 2

A long time ago, ten suns appeared in the sky.

A hero shot down nine of them with his arrows.

很久以前，天上出了十個太陽

有一個英雄用箭射下了九個太陽

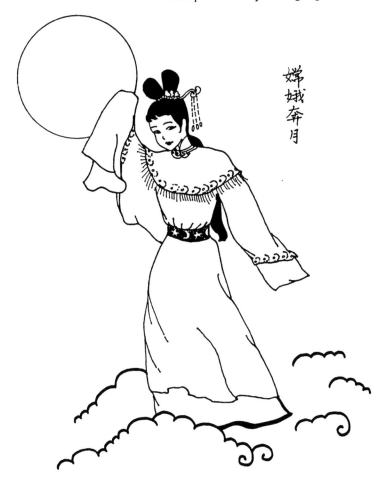

嫦娥奔月

The Heavenly Emperor gave him a special medicine that will send him soaring into the sky.

His wife, Tsang-er, ate the medicine and flew to the moon.

People admire the moon and Tsang-er during the moon festival.

天帝為了感謝他，就送他上天之之仙藥．

他的妻子嫦娥偷吃了，就飛到胱上去了．

每逢中秋節，人們乃賞月並且我朋之嫦娥．

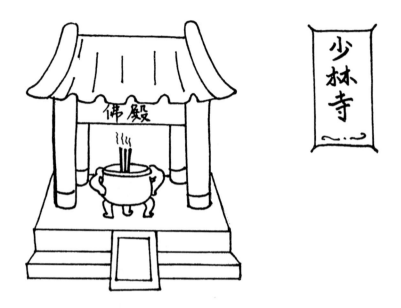

Story 3

There is a famous temple in Henan, Deng Feng.

The temple was build 1400 years ago.

在河南登封縣有了有名之少林寺.

少林寺至今己有一千四百年之歷史.

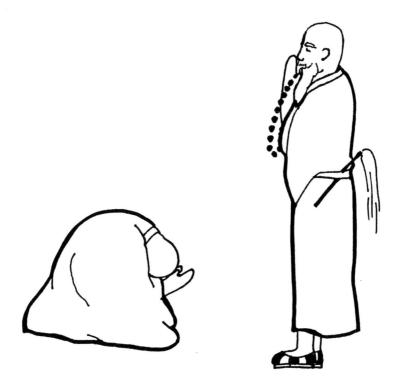

There is a tradition that the monks in the temple follow. That is the Shan-lin Kung-Fu.

Shan-lin Boxing has been passed down from generation to generation by the monks.

少林寺的和尚有練功夫之傳統.

少林拳就是少林寺和尚們傳下来的.

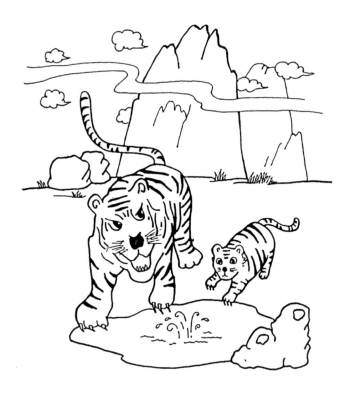

Story 4

There is a temple near the West Lake of Hong Chou.

In the temple, there is a "Tiger Dug Well."

People enjoy making tea with the water from the well.

According to legend, the well was dug out by two tigers.

在杭州西湖邊有座"虎跑寺"

寺裏有一泉井叫"虎跑泉".

人們喜歡用虎跑泉水沏茶.

傳說這泉井是由兩支老虎創洞創出來的.

Sample Informal Language Assessment Measure– Chinese

Student:_____ Date:_____

Administered by:_____

A. Answering Simple Questions

1. What is your name? 你叫什麼名字？

2. How old are you? 你今年幾歲？

3. Tell me about your family. 你家中有幾個人？

4. What is your favorite game? 你最喜歡的遊戲是什麼：

5. What did you do yesterday? 你昨天做了些什麼？

6. What did you do in school today? 你昨天在學校做了些什麼

7. When do you go to sleep? 你每天幾點睡覺？

8. What do you like to eat? 你喜歡吃什麼？

9. Where do you like to go with your family? 你喜歡跟你家人去哪裡?

10. Tell me what you watch on television. 你喜歡看什麼電視節目?

B. Following Oral Directions

1. Pick up the book. 把書拿起來.

2. Walk to the door. 走到門那邊去.

3. Put your hands under your chair. 把手放在椅子下面.

4. Put the pencil behind the box. 把鉛筆放在盒子後面.

5. Bring me a piece of paper. 拿給我一張紙.

6. Put the pencil behind your head. 把鉛筆放在頭後面.

7. Turn over the box. 把盒子翻過來.

C. Solving Problems

1. What would you do if you saw a fire? 假如你看到火, 你怎麼辦?

2. What would you do if it started raining when you were playing outside? 假如你在外面玩, 忽然下雨. 你怎麼辦?

3. What would you do if someone broke your favorite toy? 假如有一個人把你最喜歡的玩具搞壞了. 你怎麼辦?

Functional Assessment of Verbal and Nonverbal Language Behavior

Name:_____   Date of Birth:_____

Observer:_____   Home Language:_____

Informant:_____   Relationship::_____

Dates Observed:_____

	Yes	No	Frequent	Infrequent
Verbal Behavior				
1. Imitates	—	—	——	——
2. Asks questions	—	—	——	——
3. Answers	—	—	——	——
4. Requests	—	—	——	——
5. Agrees	—	—	——	——
6. Commands or directs	—	—	——	——
7. Pleads	—	—	——	——
8. Says greetings	—	—	——	——
9. Makes suggestions	—	—	——	——
10. Disagrees, argues	—	—	——	——
11. Describes objects or events	—	—	——	——
12. Describes own actions or acts	—	—	——	——
13. Describes a past experience	—	—	——	——
14. Describes future plan	—	—	——	——
15. Describes picture books, photos, etc.	—	—	——	——
16. Makes commentary	—	—	——	——
17. Protests	—	—	——	——
18. Makes promises	—	—	——	——
19. Expresses humor	—	—	——	——
20. Shows subtle hints	—	—	——	——
21. Initiates topics	—	—	——	——
22. Initiates topic shift	—	—	——	——
23. Uses compensatory strategies	—	—	——	——
24. Uses contingent query	—	—	——	——
25. Gives off-topic responses	—	—	——	——
26. Elaborates on topic already established	—	—	——	——
27. Changes speech, depending on speakers	—	—	——	——
28. Maintains topic	—	—	——	——
29. Role-plays	—	—	——	——
30. Instructs or demonstrates	—	—	——	——
31. Plans forward	—	—	——	——
32. Asks for collaborative action	—	—	——	——

	Yes	No	Frequent	Infrequent
33. Asks for clarification	—	—	————	————
34. Comments on language	—	—	————	————
35. Other	—	—	————	————

Nonverbal Behaviors

1. Head movememts
   - Nod
   - Shake
   - Tilt
   - Leans forward
2. Facial expressions
   - Smile
   - Surprise
   - Sad
   - Disgust
   - Grimace
   - Fear
   - Anger
   - Frown
   - Worry
   - Furrowed brow
   - Disbelief
   - Disagreement
3. Hand movements
   - Sign
   - Gesture
   - Point
   - Object
   - Manipulation
   - Tapping
   - Open and close fists
   - Feeling objects
   - Clasped hands
   - Wringing hands
   - Clenching fists
4. Gazing
   - Eye contact
   - Shift gaze
   - Stare
   - Look at face
   - Close eyes
   - Look down
   - Look away
5. Body movements
   - Posture shift
   - Lean forward
   - Leg/foot movements
   - Crossing and uncrossing legs
   - Rocking
   - Pacing
   - Slouching
   - Other

Bibliography

Aaronson, M., & Schaefer, E. S. (1971). Preschool preposition test. In O. G. Johnson & J. W. Bommarito (Eds.), *Tests and measurements in child development: A handbook*. San Francisco: Jossey-Bass.

Alatis, J. E. (Ed.). (1980). *Georgetown University round table on language and linguistics: Current issues in bilingual education*. Washington, DC: Georgetown University Press.

Banks, J. A. (1979). Shaping the future of multicultural education. *Journal of Negro Education, 48,* 237–253.

Bartel, N. R., & Bryen, D. N. (1978). Problems in language development. In D. D. Hamill & N. R. Bartel (Eds.), *Children with learning and behavior problems*. Boston: Allyn & Bacon.

Bedrosian, J. L. (1985). An approach to developing conversational competence. In D. N. Ripich & F. M. Spinelli (Eds.), *School discourse problems* (pp. 179–196). San Diego: College-Hill Press.

Block, L. (1972). *Facts about Filipino immigration into California*. San Francisco: R & E Research Associates.

Bloom, A. H. (1981). The linguistic shaping of thought: A study on the impact of language on thinking in China and the West. Hillsdale, NJ: Lawrence Erlbaum Associates.

Bloom, L., & Lahey, M. (1978). *Language development and language disorders*. New York: John Wiley & Sons.

Boas, F. (1946). *General anthropology*. New York: D. C. Heath.

Bowling, E. B. (1980). *Voice power*. Harrisburg, PA: Stackpole Books.

Boyle, E. (1970). *Basic course: Cantonese*. Washington, DC: U.S. Department of State.

Brooks, N. D. (1968). Teaching culture in the foreign language classroom. *Foreign Language Annals, 1,* 204–217.

Bryen, D. N. (1975). *Issues and activities in language*. Unpublished manuscript, Temple University, Philadelphia.

Buell, L. H. (1985). *Understanding the refugee ethnic Chinese*. San Diego: Los Amigos Research Associates.

California State Department of Education, Office of Bilingual Bicultural Education. (1981). *Schooling and language minority students: A theoretical framework*. Los Angeles: Evaluation, Dissemination and Assessment Center, California State University.

California State Department of Education. (1983). *A handbook for teaching Korean-speaking students*. Sacramento: Author.

California State Department of Education. (1984a). *A handbook for teaching Cantonese-speaking students*. Sacramento: Author.

California State Department of Education. (1984b). *A handbook for teaching Vietnamese-speaking students*. Sacramento: Author.

California State Department of Education. (1984c). *A handbook on California education for language minority parents*. Sacramento: Author.

Canale, M. (1981). From communicative competence to communicative language pedagogy. In J. Richard & R. Schmidt (Eds.), *Language and communication* New York: Longman.

Canale, M., & Swain, M. (1980). Theoretical bases of communicative approaches to second language teaching and testing. *Applied Linguistics, 1*, 1–47.

Carrow, E. (1974). *Carrow elicited language inventory*. Austin, TX: Learning Concepts.

Cazden, C. (1972). *Child language and education*. New York: Holt, Rinehart & Winston.

Cazden, C., & Hymes, D. (1972). *Functions of language in the classroom*. New York: Teachers College Press.

Center for Applied Linguistics. (1981). *Language in education: Theory and practice*. Washington, DC: Author.

Center for Applied Linguistics, Clearinghouse on Language and Linguistics. (1981). *Indochinese students in U.S. schools: A guide for administrators*. Washington, DC: Author.

Chandler, M. J., Greenspan, S., & Barenboim, C. (1974). Assessment and training of role-taking and referential communication skills in institutionalized emotionally disturbed children. *Developmental Psychology*.

Chang, R., & Chang, M. S. (1978). *Speaking of Chinese*. New York: W. W. Norton.

Chen, M. (1985). Three presentations of two semantically equivalent passages. Lecture delivered at San Diego State University.

Cheng, L. L. (1983). *An ethnographic study of language-impaired preschoolers*. Unpublished doctoral dissertation, San Diego.

Chin, T. (Ed.). (1967). *A history of the Chinese in California*. San Francisco: Chinese History Society of America.

Chomsky, N. (1965). *Aspects of the theory of syntax*. Cambridge, MA: MIT Press.

Chu-Chang, M. (1981). The dependency relation between oral language and reading in bilingual children. *Journal of Education, 163*(1).

Chun, J. (1980, Fall). A survey of research in second language acquisition. *Modern Language Journal*, 296–297.

Cook-Gumperz, J. (1978, October). Communicating with young children in the home. *Theory into Practice*.

Cook-Gumperz, J., & Gumperz, J. J. (1979). *Beyond ethnography: Some uses of sociolinguistics for understanding classroom environments*. Paper presented at the American Education Research Association Conference, San Francisco.

Corder, S. P. (1967). The significance of learner's errors. *International Review of Applied Linguistics in Language Teaching, 5*, 162–169.

Cummins, J. (1978). Bilingualism and the development of metalinguistic awareness. *Journal of Cross-Cultural Psychology, 9*, 131–149.

Cummins, J. (1981). The role of primary language development in promoting educational success for language minority students. In California State Department of Education, Office of Bilingual Bicultural Education (Ed.), *Schooling and language minority students: A theoretical framework*. Los Angeles: Evaluation, Dissemination and Assessment Center, California State University.

Data/Bical Reports. Sacramento: California State Department of Education Bilingual Office.

Davie, M. R. (1974). *Refugees in America*. New York: Harper & Row.

Dickson, W. P. (1982). Creating communication-rich classrooms: Insights from the sociolinguistic and referential traditions. In L. C. Wilkinson (Ed.), *Communicating in the classroom*. New York: Academic Press.

Douglass, M. (1981). Introduction to the yearbook. *Claremont Reading Conference 45th Yearbook*. Claremont.

Dowling B. T., Hendricks, G., Mason, S., & Olney, D. (1984). Hmong resettlement. *Cura Reporter, 14*(3), 1–8.

Dulay, H., & Burt, M. (1972). Goofing: An indicator of children's second language learning strategies. *Language Learning, 22*, 235–251.

Dulay, H. C., & Burt, M. K. (1977). Remarks on creativity in second language acquisition. In M. K. Burt, H. C. Dulay, & M. Finnochiaro (Eds.), *Viewpoints on English as a second language*, (pp. 95–126). New York: Regents.

Emerick, L., & Hatten, L. (1979). *Diagnosis and evaluation in speech pathology*. Englewood Cliffs, NJ: Prentice-Hall.

Erickson, F. (1978). *On standards of descriptive validity in studies of classroom activities*. Paper presented at the American Education Research Association Conference, Toronto, Canada.

Ervin-Tripp, S. (1969). Commentary on a paper by R. M. Jones. In L. G. Kelley (Ed.), *Description and measurement of bilingualism: An international seminar*. Toronto: University of Toronto Press.

Ervin-Tripp, S. (1974). Is second language learning like the first? *TESOL Quarterly, 8*, 137–144.

Fillmore, C. J., Kempler, D., & Wong, S. Y. (1979). *Individual differences in language ability and behavior*. New York: Academic Press.

Fillmore, L. W. (1984). *Variations in second language acquisitions: What is normal and what is not?* Paper presented at the conference of the American Speech-Language-Hearing Association, San Francisco.

Frake, C. (1964). A structural description of Subanun religious behavior. In W. Goodenough (Ed.), *Explorations in cultural anthropology*. New York: McGraw-Hill.

Frazer, J. G. (1964). *Totemism and exogamy*. London.

Fromkin, V., & Rodman, R. (1974). *An introduction to language*. New York: Holt, Rinehart & Winston.

Gallagher, T., & Prutting, C. (1983). *Pragmatic assessment and intervention issues in language*. San Diego: College-Hill Press.

Gardner, H. (1983). *Frames of mind*. New York: Basic Books.

Garkovitch, L. E. (1977). *The Indochinese refugee: A critique of assimilation theories*. Paper presented at the annual meeting of the Midwest Sociological Society, Minneapolis.

Genesee, F. (1978). Is there an optimal age for starting second language instruction? *McGill Journal of Education, 13*, 145–154.

Goodman, K. (1976). Manifesto for a reading revolution. *Claremont Reading Conference 40th Yearbook*. Claremont.

Gordon, M. M. (1978). *Human nature, class and ethnicity*. New York: Oxford University Press.

Gordon, M. M. (1964). *Assimilation in American life*. New York: Oxford University Press.

Grant, M. (1919). *The passing of the great race*. New York: Charles Scribner's Sons.

Greenfield, P. M., & Smith, J. H. (1976). *Communication and the beginning of language: The development of syntactic structure in one-word speech and beyond*. New York: Academic Press.

Groff, P. (1977). Oral language and reading. *Reading World, 17*.

Gumperz, J. (1971). *Language in social groups*. Stanford: Stanford University Press.

Gumperz, J. (1982). *Discourse strategies*. Cambridge, England: Cambridge University Press.

Halliday, M. A. K. (1975). *Explorations in the function of language*. London: Edward Arnold.

Halliday, M. A. K. (1975). *Learning how to mean*. New York: Elsevier North-Holland.

Halliday, M. A. K. (1978). *Language as social semiotic*. Baltimore: University Park Press.

Heath, S. B. (1983). *Ways with words—Language, life, and work in communities and classrooms*. Cambridge, England: Cambridge University Press.

Heath, S. B. (1985). *Second language acquisitions*. Paper presented at the conference of the American Speech-Language-Hearing Association, San Francisco, CA.

Hunsaker, P. L., & Allessandra, A. J. (1980). *The art of managing people*. Englewood Cliffs, NJ: Prentice-Hall.

Hylteenstam, K., & Peinemann, M. (1985). *Modeling and assessing second language acquisition*. San Diego: College-Hill Press.

Hymes, D. (1971). *On communicative competence*. Philadelphia: University of Pennsylvania Press.

Hymes, D. (1974). *Foundations in sociolinguistics*. Philadelphia: University of Pennsylvania Press.

Iglesias, A. (1985). Cultural conflict in the classroom: The communicatively different child. In D. N. Ripich & F. M. Spinelli (Eds.), *School discourse problems* (pp. 79–96). San Diego: College-Hill Press.

Kallen, H. M. (1924). *Culture and democracy in the United States.* New York: Boni and Liveright.

Kallen, H. M. (1956). *Cultural pluralism and the American idea.* Philadelphia: University of Pennsylvania Press.

Kent, D. P. (1953). The refugee intellectual. New York: Columbia University Press.

Kessler, C. (1971). *The acquisition of syntax in bilingual child.* Washington, DC: Georgetown University Press.

Kiraithe, J. M. (1985, December). *Second language acquisition: Implications for assessment and placement.* Paper presented at the Conference of Special Education and the Bilingual Child, Pasadena, CA.

Kluckhohn, C. & Kelly, W. H. (1945). The concept of culture. In R. Linton (Ed.), *Science of man in the world crisis.* New York: Columbia University Press.

Krashen, S. D. (1978). Second language acquisition. In W. O. Dingwall (Ed.), *A survey of linguistic science* (2nd ed., pp. 317–338). Stamford, CT: Greylord.

Krashen, S. D. (1981). Bilingual education and second language acquisition theory. In California State Department of Education, Office of Bilingual Bicultural Education (Ed.), *Schooling and language minority students: A theoretical framework.* Los Angeles: Evaluation, Dissemination and Assessment Center, California State University.

Krashen, S. D., Long, M. A., & Scarcella, R. C. (1979). Age, rate and eventual attainment in second language acquisition. *TESOL Quarterly, 13*(4), 5735–5782.

Kroeber, A. L. (1952). *The nature of culture.* Chicago: University of Chicago Press.

Kroeber, A. L., & Kluckhohn, C. (1954). *Culture: A critical review of concepts and definitions.* New York: Random House.

Krug, M. M. (1976). *Cultural pluralism in a historical perspective* (Occasional Paper). San Diego State University, Institute for Cultural Pluralism, San Diego.

Lado, R. (1957). *Linguistics across cultures.* Ann Arbor: University of Michigan Press.

Lenneberg, E. (1967). *Biological foundations of language.* New York: John Wiley & Sons.

Leonard, L. B. (1979). Language impairment in children. *Merrill-Palmer Quarterly, 25.*

Leonard, L. B., Perrozzi, J. A., Prutting, C. A., & Berkeley, R. K. (1978). Nonstandardized approaches to the assessment of language behaviors. *ASHA, 20.*

Lim, H. S. (1978). A study of Korean-American cultural relations. *Korean Journal, 18*(6).

Linfors, J. (1980). *Children's language and learning.* Englewood Cliffs, NJ: Prentice-Hall.

Liu, W. T., & Yu, E. S. H. (1975). Asian-American youth. In R. J. Havighurst, P. H. Dreyer, & K. V. Rehage (Eds.), *Youth* (pp. 367–389). Chicago: National Society for the Study of Education.

Loban, W. (1963). *The language of elementary school children* (NCTE Report No. 1). Urbana, IL: National Council of Teachers of English.

Lund, N. J., & Duchan, J. F. (1983). *Assessing children's language in naturalistic contexts.* Englewood Cliffs, NJ: Prentice-Hall.

Mandelbaum, D. G. (1949). *Selected writings of Edward Sapir.* Berkeley: University of California Press.

McClatchy, V. S. (1972). *Japanese immigration and colonization.* San Francisco: R & E Research Associates.

McCunn, R. L. (1979). *An illustrated history of the Chinese in America.* San Francisco: Design Enterprises of San Francisco.

McLaughlin, B. (1978). *Second language acquisition in childhood.* New York: John Wiley & Sons.

Mehan, H. (1978). Structuring school structures. *Harvard Education Review.*

Menyuk, P. (1971). *The acquisition and development of language.* Englewood Cliffs, NJ: Prentice-Hall.

Meredith, W., & Cramer, S. (1982). Hmong refugees in Nebraska. In B. Downing & D. Olney (Eds.), *The Hmong in the west: Observations and reports* (pp. 353–362). Minneapolis, MN: Southeast Asian Refugee Studies Project, Center for Urban and Regional Affairs, University of Minnesota.

Miramontes, O. (1984, November). *Miscue analysis of Hispanic primary and secondary readers: Implication for transition into English.* Paper presented at the meeting of the American Anthropological Association, Denver, CO.

Miyawaki, K., et al. (1975). An effect of linguistic experience: The discrimination of [r] and [l] by native speakers of Japanese and English. *Perception and Psychophysics, 18,* 331–340.

Monane, T. A. (1978). Producing effective bilinguals: Language classroom techniques to facilitate codeswitching within the socio-semantic contexts of everyday life. *Georgetown University round table on languages and linguistics.* Washington, DC: Georgetown University Press.

Moulton, R. (1554). *China: A world apart.* Presented at the American Speech-Language-Hearing Association Convention, San Francisco.

Nguyen, L. T., & Henkin, A.B. (1953). Change among Indochinese refugees. In R. J. Samuda & S. C. Woods (Eds.) Perspectives in immigrant and minority education. New York: University Press of America.

Ochs, E., & Schieffelin, B. (1979). *Developmental pragmatics.* New York: Academic Press.

Ojemann, G. A., & Whitaker, H. A. (1978). The bilingual brain. *Archives of Neurology, 35,* 410-412.

Philips, S. (1983). *The invisible culture.* New York: Longman.

Piaget, J. (1972). Language and thought from the genetic point of view. In A. Parveen (Ed.), *Language and thinking.* Middlesex, England: Penguin Books.

Prizant, B. (1978). *An analysis of functions of immediate echolalia in autistic children.* Unpublished doctoral dissertation, State University of New York, Buffalo.

Prutting, C. A. (1982). Pragmatics as social competence. *Journal of Speech and Hearing Disorders, 47,* 123–133.

Prutting, C. A., & Kirchner, D. M. (1983). Applied pragmatics. In T. M. Gallagher & C. A. Prutting (Eds.), *Pragmatic assessment and intervention issues in language.* San Diego: College-Hill Press.

Ripich, D. N., & Spinelli, F. M. (1985). An ethnographic approach to assessment and intervention. In D. N. Ripich & F. M. Spinelli (Eds.), *School discourse problems* (pp. 199–217). San Diego: College-Hill Press.

Rosansky, E. (1975). The critical period for the acquisition of language: Some cognitive developmental considerations. *Working Papers on bilingualism, 6,* 92–102.

Ruddel, R. (1967). Oral language and the development of other language skills. In W. T. Petty (Ed.), *Research in oral language.* Urbana, IL: National Council of Teachers of English.

San Diego County Department of Education. (1981). *Bilingual-bicultural assistance to special education.* San Diego: Author.

Sapir, E. (1921). *Language: An Introduction to the study of speech.* New York: Harcourt, Brace & Company.

Sasanuma, S. (1974). Impairment of written language in Japanese aphasics: Kana versus kanji processing. *Journal of Chinese Linguistics, 2,* 141–158.

Shuy, R. W. (1978). In J. E. Alatis (Ed.), *Bilingualism and language variety.* Washington DC: Georgetown University Press.

Simon, C. (1979). Philosophy for learning disabled children: Thinking. *Journal of Child Psychology, 1*(1).

Slobin, D. (1973). Cognitive prerequisites for the development of grammar. In C. Ferguson & D. Slobin (Eds.), *Studies of child language development.* New York: Holt, Rinehart & Winston.

Smalley, W. A. (1984). Adaptive language strategies of the Hmong: From Asian mountains to American ghettos. *Language Science, 7*(2), 241–269.

Smith, F. (1982). *How children learn? Interdisciplinary Voice No. 1.* Austin, TX: Society for Learning Disabilities and Remedial Education.

Snow, C. (1977). The development of conversation between mothers and babies. *Journal of Language, 4.*

Spencer, H. (1888). *The principle of sociology* (pp. 435–459).

Spencer, P. (1970). *Reading.* Alpha Iota Chapter of Di Lambda Theta, Claremont, CA: Claremont Graduate School.

Spencer, P. (1977). Reading is creative living. *Claremont Reading Conference 21st Yearbook,* Claremont, CA.

Stephens, W. D. (1970). *California and the Orientals.* San Francisco: R & E Research Associates.

Taylor, B. (1974). Toward a theory of language acquisition. *Language Learning, 24,* 23–36.

Taylor, O. (1986). *Treatment of Communication Disorders in Culturally & Linguistically Diverse Populations.* San Diego: College-Hill Press.

Taylor, O. & Payne, K. (1983). Culturally valid testing: A proactive approach, *Topics in Learning Disorders, 3* 8–20.

Tè, H. D. (1984). *Contrastive Analysis of English & Vietnamese Vowel & Consonant Systems.* (Unpublished Paper).

Thuy, V. G. (1983). The Indochinese in America: Who are they and how are they doing? In D. T. Nakanishi & M. Hirano-Nakanishi (Eds.). *The education of Asian and Pacific Americans: Historical perspectives and prescription for the future* (pp. 103–121). Phoenix, AZ: Oryx Press.

Toukomaa, P., & Stutnabb-Kangas, T. (1977). *The intensive teaching of the mother tongue to migrant children of preschool age and children in the lower level of comprehensive school* (Research Report No. 26). Tampere, Finland: Department of Sociology and Social Psychology, University of Tampere, Finland.

Trueba, H. T. (1983). Adjustment problems of Mexican and Mexican-American students: An anthropological study. *Learning Disability Quarterly, 6*(4), 395–415.

Trueba, H. T. (1984). Organizing classroom instruction in specific sociocultural contexts: Teaching Mexican youth to write.

Trueba, H. T., & Wright, P. (1980–1981). On ethnographic studies and multicultural education. *Journal of the National Association for Bilingual Education, 5*(2).

Tse, J. (1980). A descriptive analysis of three aspects of tone changes from middle to modern Chinese. *Studies in English Literature and Linguistics.*

Tylor, E. B. (1871). *Primitive Culture.* New York: Gordon Press.

Tzeng, O. J. L., & Wang, W. S. Y. (1983). The first two R's. *American Scientist, 71,* 238–243.

Utah test of language disorders. (1977). Salt Lake City: Communication Research Associates.

Uzgiris, I., & Hunt, J. (1975). *Assessment in infancy.* Urbana: University of Illinois.

Van Riper, C. (1963). *Speech correction: Principles and methods.* Englewood Cliffs, NJ: Prentice-Hall.

Vygotsky, L. (1962). *Thought and language.* Cambridge, MA: MIT Press.

Walfram, W. A. (1976). Levels of sociolinguistic bias in testing. In D. S. Harrison & T. Trabass (Eds). *Black English: A Seminar.* Hillsdale, NJ: Lawrence Erlbaum Associates.

Walfram, W. A. (1983). Test interpretation and sociolinguistic differences. *Topics in Language Disorders, 3,* 8–20.

Walker, C. L. (1985). Learning English: The Southeast Asia refugee experience. *Topics in Language Disorders, 5* (4), 53–65.

Wang, W. S. Y. (1967). Phonological features of tone. *IJAL, 33.*

Wang, W. S. Y. (1983). Speech and script relations in some Asian languages. In M. Chu-Chang & V. Rodriguez (Eds.), *Asian and Pacific-American perspective in bilingual education.* New York: Teachers College Press.

Warner, W. L., & Srole, L. (1945). *The Social System of American Ethnic Groups.* New Haven: Yale University Press.

Wei, T. T. D. (1983). The Vietnamese refugee child: Understanding cultural differences. In D. R. Omark & J. G. Erickson (Eds.), *The bilingual exceptional child* (pp. 197–212). San Diego: College-Hill Press.

Wilkinson, A. M. (1967, October). Oracy in English teaching. *Elementary English, 45.*

Wilkinson, L. L., & Spinelli, F. (1982). In L. L. Wilkinson (Ed.), *Communicating in the classroom.* New York: Academic Press.

Wilson, S. (1977). The use of ethnographic techniques in educational research. *Review of Educational Research, 17*(1), 245–265.

Wong, Y. M. (1983). *Dear Diane: Letters from our daughters.* Oakland, CA: Asian Women United of California.

Wong-Fillmore, L. (1985). Learning a second language: Chinese children in the American classroom. In J. E. Alatis & J. J. Staczek (Eds.), *Perspectives on bilingualism and bilingual education* (pp. 436–452). Washington, DC: Georgetown University Press.

Wong-Fillmore L. (1985). When does teacher talk work as input. In S. M. Gass & C. G. Madden (Eds.), *Input in second language acquisition,* (pp. 15–50). Rowley, MA: Newbury House.

Wong-Fillmore, L., Ammon, P., Ammon, M. S., DeLucchi, K., Jensen, J., McLaughlin, B., & Strong, M. (1983). *Learning language through bilingual instruction: Second year report.* University of California, National Institute of Education.

Yeh, T. M. (1982). *Drill exercises in Mandarin pronunciation.* Taipei: National Taiwan University.

Zangwill, I. (1910). *The melting pot.* New York: Macmillan Co.

Zimmerman, I., Steiner, V., & Pond, R. E. (1979). *Preschool language scale.* Columbus: Charles E. Merrill Publishing Co.

Additional Tests and Other Educational Tools

Native Language Proficiency Tests

Babel Chinese Proficiency Test. A test of proficiency in Chinese. B.A.B.E.L. Inc., 255 East 14th St., Oakland, CA 94606.

Basic Elementary Skills Test (BEST). A test of basic elementary skills in Chinese, Vietnamese and Cambodian. Los Amigos Research Associates, 7035 Galewood, San Diego, CA 92120.

Bilingual Syntax Measure—Tagalog (BSM-T). A test of language dominance for Tagalog speakers. Asian-American Bilingual Center, Berkeley Unified School District, Berkeley, CA.

Bilingual Syntax Measure—Chinese (BSM-C). A test of language dominance for speakers of Chinese. Asian-American Bilingual Center, Berkeley Unified School District, Berkeley, CA.

Cantonese Test 1. A test of oral skills for Cantonese speakers. Oakland Unified School District, 1025 Second Ave., Oakland, CA 94606.

Chinese Oral Proficiency Test. A test of oral proficiency in Chinese. B.A.B.E.L. Inc., 255 East 14th St., Oakland, CA 94606.

Chinese Test. Chinese Literature & Cultural Test. Chinese Bilingual Test. Antoinette Metcalf. Test and materials for use with speakers of Chinese. AB893 Chinese Bilingual Project, San Francisco Unified School District, San Francisco, CA.

Criterion-Referenced Test for Golden-Mountain Reading Series—Chinese. A criteria-referenced test for speakers of Chinese. Suitable for grades 1 to 6. San Francisco Unified School District, 950 Clay St., San Francisco, CA 94108.

Daly City Oral Language Survey—Tagalog. A descriptive survey to monitor progress of Tagalog speakers. Suitable for grades K to 3. Jefferson School District, 101 Lincoln Ave., Daly City, CA 94015.

Home Language Questionnaire—Chinese, Vietnamese and Tagalog. Questionnaire to survey the use of home language. Suitable for grades K to 12. B.A.B.E.L., 255 East 14th St., Oakland, CA 94606.

Marysville Test of Language Dominance—Tagalog. A test of language proficiency for Tagalog speakers. Suitable for grades K to 5. Marysville Reading Learning Center, 11th and Powerline, Oliverhurst, CA 95961.

MAT—SEA—CAL Oral Proficiency Tests—Chinese, Tagalog, Mandarin, Cantonese. A test to determine needs for remedial instruction. Suitable for grades K to 5. Center for Applied Linguistics, 1611 North Kent St., Arlington, Va 22209.

Multicultural Vocabulary Test. A test of vocabulary using body parts as stimulus items. Suitable for different ages. Los Amigos Research Associates, 7035 Galewood, San Diego, CA 92120.

Short Test of Linguistic Skills (STLS—Chinese, Vietnamese, Tagalog). A descriptive test of expressive language skills. Suitable for grades 3 to 7. Chicago Board of Education, 2021 N. Burling St., Chicago, IL 60611.

SWCEL Test of Oral Language Proficiency—Chinese. A test to assess the need for remedial instruction. Southwestern Cooperative Educational Laboratory, Inc., 229 Traman, N.E., Albuquerque, NM 87108.

Bicultural/Multicultural References

Cassettes on Cultural Diversity. Perspectives on education, learning styles, family, culture, and social values of different cultural groups: Indian, Spanish, Asian American, Black Children. The Council for Exceptional Children, 1920 Association Dr., Reston, VA 22091.

Chinese Bilingual Bicultural Enrichment Test. A test of cultural awareness. Oakland Unified School District, 1025 Second Ave., Oakland, CA 94606.

Education of Culturally and Linguistically Different Exceptional Children. A collection of research-based papers to serve the professional. Contains information on bilingual and culturally different exceptional children. Edited by Philip C. Chinn. Council for Exceptional Children, Dept. BLN, 1920 Association Dr., Reston, VA 22091.

Human Services for Cultural Minorities. Richard H. Dana. Investigates the values, beliefs, and continuing cultural practices of Native Americans, Afro-Americans, Hispanic Americans and Asian Americans. Pro Ed, 5341 Industrial Oaks Blvd., Austin, TX 78735.

Refugee Update. A newsletter about refugees. Folsom Cordona Unified School District, Folsom, CA 95630.

Language Materials and Bilingual Materials. A survey of materials for the study of the uncommonly taught languages. This series includes 8 annotated bibliographies on uncommonly taught languages from Western Europe; Eastern Europe and the Soviet Union; the Middle East and North Africa; southern Asia; eastern Asia; Sub-Sahara Africa; Southeast Asia and the Pacific; North, Central and South America. Center for Applied Linguistics Publications, 3520 Prospect St., NW, Washington, DC 20001.

Bilingual Materials Catalog (Chinese, Vietnamese, Philipino, Cambodian). Contains instructional materials. The National Hispanic University, 255 East 14th St., Oakland, CA 94606.

Cambodian/English Illustrated Vocabulary, Level 1. Vietnamese/English Illustrated Vocabulary, Levels I, II, III. Contains illustrations and terminology related to such concepts as the human body, family, home, people, school, transportation, nature, alphabet, numbers, and others. Level I is useful for beginners of any age level. Levels II and III contain more key words and emphasize survival language skills. B.A.B.E.L. Inc., 255 East 14th St., Oakland, CA 94606.

Cassette Tapes. A colloquium on Vietnamese. How to Teach ESL. Eng-Khmer phrasebook for Cambodians. Eng-Lao phrasebook for Laotians. Center of Applied Linguistics Publications, 3520 Prospect St., NW, Washington, DC 20001.

Dara Reads Lao. Multifunctional Support Service Center, San Diego State University, San Diego, CA 92182.

From the Dragon's Cloud. A collection of Vietnamese folk tales in English. Center for Applied Linguistics Publications, 3520 Prospect NW, Washington, DC 20001.

Vietnamese Educational Materials. English-Viet phrasebook for Vietnamese and accompanying cassettes. Viet-English Phrasebook for English and accompanying cassettes. Handbook for teachers, selected bibliography for teaching English to Vietnamese. Center for Applied Linguistics Publications, 3520 Prospect St., NW, Washington, DC 20001.

Vietnamese Curriculum Materials. Curriculum materials for use with the Vietnamese population. Consult publisher for catalog. Developmental Learning Materials, 6504 Tracor Lane, Austin, TX 78721.

Workbook on Pilipino—Level I. Bilingual (English/Pilipino) workbook. B.A.B.E.L. Inc., 255 East 14th St., Oakland, CA 94606.

Foreign Accent

Compton Phonological Assessment of Foreign Accent. Assessment of English Phonology. Arthur J. Compton, Carousel House, P.O. Box 4480, San Francisco, CA 94101.

Foreign Accent Improvement Series. Pronouncing ESL for Cantonese, Filipino, Japanese, Korean, Mandarin, Vietnamese. Articulation programs utilizing cassette practice tapes. Arthur J. Compton, Carousel House, P.O. Box 4480, San Francisco, CA 94101.

Miscellaneous

Tips for Talking to the Hard of Hearing. One page illustrated tips for the hard-of-hearing available in English, Cambodian, Chinese, Portuguese, Vietnamese, Japanese, and Tagalog. Hearing Society for the Bay Area, Inc., 1428 Bush St., San Francisco, CA 94109.

Glossary

ABC American-born Chinese.

affective filter the effect of personality, motivation, and other "affective variables" on second language acquisition.

ASHA American Speech-Language-Hearing Association.

baci a religious ceremony performed by some Indochinese (specifically Laotians) for healing purposes or celebration.

BICS basic interpersonal communication skills; the aspects of language proficiency strongly associated with the basic communication fluency achieved by all normal native speakers of a language.

bilingual a person who has skills in two languages, although not necessarily equal for both languages.

CALP cognitive academic linguistic proficiency; the aspects of language proficiency strongly related to literacy and academic achievement.

code switching a change in the target language during the course of a conversation.

communicative competence mastery of the language code, the appropriate language use in different sociolinguistic contexts, ways to combine meanings and forms to achieve a unified text in different modes, and the verbal and nonverbal strategies to compensate for communication breakdowns and to enhance effective communication.

comprehensible input message that the language learner understands.

contrastive studies/error analysis the comparison of two linguistic systems (L1 and L2) in terms of phonological, morphological, syntactical, and semantic features to look for fundamental differences and to define problems that speakers of L1 are likely to have in learning L2.

discourse analysis the study of communicative interaction between the L2 learner and his or her interactants.

ESL English as a second language.

ethnography the methods of study of events, persons, and interaction that enable researchers to ascertain the underlying rules that operate for the participants.

FEP fluent English proficiency.

FES fluent English-speaking.

GRE Graduate Record Examination.

Hiragana cursive Japanese writing system.

interference the errors made by someone learning a new language in the transition from one phonological system to another.

interlanguage the intermediate step between a language learner's native and target languages. It is a unique system, distinct from L1 and L2.

I/T interpreter/translator.

Kanji the Chinese characters used in the Japanese writing system.

Karma a word used in the Indian religion to mean "fate."

Katakana Japanese writing system.

kinesics gestures; body movements, including facial expressions; posture; eye and head movements.

L1 first language.

L2 second language.

LEA local education agency.

LEP limited English proficiency.

LES limited English speaking.

limited bilingualism low skill levels in two languages.

marginal the quality of being caught between the values and norms of the host society and those of the native culture, resulting in a state of double cultural orientation.

metalinguistics comments on language as seen in language games, vocal play, use of jokes or figurative language.

mixing the intra- and intersentential intermingling of native and second language features.

morpheme studies the investigation of L2 learners' acquisition of grammatical morphemes in order to identify whether an invariant order of morpheme acquisition was parallel to what had been found in L1 context.

NEP non-English proficiency.

NES non–English-speaking.

PALI the Pacific and Asian Linguistics Institutes of the University of Hawaii.

paralanguage prosodic features such as pitch, stress, intonation; backchanneling; other oral, but nonverbal behaviors.

partial bilingualism skill in two languages, but nativelike proficiency in only one.

participant observation a term used by anthropologists meaning "doing ethnography" by observing and noting the activation of the participants.

pidgin (*pigeon*) a form of speech that usually has a simplified grammar and limited and often mixed vocabulary. The word *business* was misproduced and sounded like "pidgin" to the Chinese.

proficient bilingualism nativelike skills in two languages.

proxemics the perception and use of social and personal space, as well as the use of space boundaries, in interpersonal communication.

SEA state education agency.

sequential second language the adding of a second language once the learner has a good first language.

shift a move from mother tongue to the new language as the language of primary use.

silent period a time during which language learners are building up competence via input, by listening.

simultaneous second language acquisition bilingual acquisition of two languages in very young children.

sociosemantic context the social situations of everyday life and the communication of meanings that are relevant to these social situations.

turn-taking the exchange between the participants of a conversation.

transfer influence of the first language (L1) upon second language (L2).

variability analysis the use of the inconsistency of the L2 learners' output to make inferences about the L2 learners' interlanguage competence.

Index

H

I

J

K

L

M

N

T

U

V

W